CHAIR EXERCISES FOR SENIORS SIMPLIFIED

THE ILLUSTRATED BEGINNER'S GUIDE TO IMPROVE YOUR BALANCE AND MOBILITY WITH EASY YOGA AND STRENGTH ROUTINES

INSIGHT EDITIONS

CONTENTS

Introduction 7

1. UNDERSTANDING CHAIR EXERCISES 9
1.1 What are Chair Exercises? Defining Your Path to Mobility 9
1.2 The Top 5 Benefits of Chair Exercises for Seniors 11
1.3 Safety First: Preparing Your Space and Choosing the Right Chair 13

2. OVERCOMING COMMON BARRIERS 17
2.1 Navigating Limited Mobility: Exercises Tailored for All Abilities 17
2.2 Easing Fears: Injury Prevention through Proper Technique 19
2.3 Making Exercise Accessible: Solutions for Vision and Space Limitations 21

3. SETTING UP FOR SUCCESS 25
3.1 Equipment Essentials: Simplifying Your Exercise Toolkit 25
3.2 Personalizing Your Routine: Listening to Your Body's Needs 28
3.3 Staying Motivated: Setting Realistic Goals and Tracking Progress 30

4. ENHANCING STRENGTH AND MUSCLE TONE 33
4.1 Arm Strength: Using Resistance Bands for Toning 33
4.2 Core Stability: Safe Exercises to Strengthen Your Abdominals 38
4.3 Leg and Glute Workouts: Building Lower Body Strength 42

5. IMPROVING FLEXIBILITY AND BALANCE 47
5.1 Gentle Stretching: A Guide to Increased Flexibility 47
5.2 Balance in a Chair: Exercises to Find Your Center 50
5.3 Dynamic Movements for Everyday Stability 52

6. CHAIR YOGA FOR MIND AND BODY   55
   6.1 Breathing Techniques: The Foundation of
   Chair Yoga   55
   6.2 Relaxation and Meditation: Mindful Movements
   in a Chair   58
   6.3 Yoga Poses Adapted for Chair Practice   60

7. BOOSTING CARDIOVASCULAR HEALTH   73
   7.1 The Joy of Chair Marching: An Introduction to
   Cardio   73
   7.2 Seated Dance Moves: Combining Fun and Fitness   78
   7.3 Cardio Circuit: Rotating Through Heart-Healthy
   Exercises   80

8. TAILORING EXERCISES FOR HEALTH
  CONDITIONS   85
   8.1 Chair Exercises for Those with Arthritis   85
   8.2 Safe Movements for Seniors with Osteoporosis   88
   8.3 Cardio Routines for Heart Health   90

9. CHAIR EXERCISES FOR WHEELCHAIR USERS   95
   9.1 Upper Body Strength and Flexibility for
   Wheelchair Users   95
   9.2 Core Exercises Adapted for Wheelchair Stability   98

10. ADVANCED CHAIR EXERCISE TECHNIQUES   101
   10.1 Increasing Exercise Intensity Safely   101
   10.2 Combining Movements for Compound
   Workouts   104
   10.3 Integrating Small Weights for Added Resistance 106

11. PAIN MANAGEMENT AND INJURY PREVENTION   109
   11.1 Listening to Your Body: Recognizing Good Pain
   vs. Bad Pain   109
   11.2 Warm-Up and Cool-Down: Essential for Injury
   Prevention   112
   11.3 Addressing Common Exercise Related Aches   114

12. NUTRITION AND HYDRATION   117
   12.1 Eating for Strength: Nutritional Guidelines for
   Seniors   117
   12.2 Staying Hydrated: The Role of Water in Senior
   Health   120

13. THE ROLE OF SLEEP IN RECOVERY 123
    13.1 Optimizing Your Sleep for Better Health 123
    13.2 Creating a Restful Environment: Tips for Seniors 126

14. THE MENTAL AND EMOTIONAL BENEFITS OF CHAIR EXERCISES 129
    14.1 Exercise as Stress Relief: The Psychological Upsides 129
    14.2 Building Confidence and Independence Through Movement 131
    14.3 The Social Aspect: Connecting with Others Through Exercise 133

15. CREATING A ROUTINE THAT LASTS 137
    15.1 Daily Habits for Long-Term Success 137
    15.2 Mixing It Up: How to Keep Chair Exercises Fresh and Engaging 140
    15.3 Setting and Adjusting Goals Over Time 142

16. LEVERAGING TECHNOLOGY FOR SUPPORT 145
    16.1 Fitness Apps and Trackers: Your Digital Companions 145
    16.2 Finding Online Support Groups and Virtual Classes 148

17. CONTINUING YOUR JOURNEY BEYOND THE CHAIR 151
    17.1 From Chair to Life: Translating Exercise into Everyday Activities 151
    17.2 Exploring New Hobbies with Renewed Energy 154
    17.3 Volunteering: Giving Back with Your Gained Strength and Mobility 157
    17.4 Setting New Horizons: Goals Beyond Chair Exercises 159

    Conclusion 163
    Resources 165

INTRODUCTION

As we age, each step and movement can feel like a challenge. Simple daily living that we once took for granted—climbing stairs and getting out of a car—can become daunting. But what if there was a way to reclaim your mobility and enhance your independence, all from the safety and comfort of a chair?

My journey into the world of fitness was born out of necessity. After both hip and knee replacements, I found myself struggling with traditional exercises. I needed something that respected my body's limits and challenged it to improve. That's when I discovered chair exercises—a transformative practice that catered to my fitness level and significantly enhanced my strength and flexibility.

This book is a culmination of all I have learned and experienced. The book is designed to help you engage in physical activity that is both doable and effective, regardless of your current fitness abilities. The goal is simple: to improve your balance, mobility, and overall health, thereby boosting your independence and quality of life.

You will find that this guide breaks down each exercise into easy-to-follow steps with accompanying illustrations that make starting any routine a breeze. Whether it's yoga to enhance your flexibility or strength routines to build muscle, each category is tailored to meet your needs. I've also included advice on selecting the right equipment and tailoring exercises to accommodate various health conditions.

This book is designed to be inclusive and accessible. It addresses all seniors, including those who may use a wheelchair, with large print, clear images, and a friendly narrative style that makes each page inviting and easy to understand. From foundational exercises to more advanced techniques and extending into essential lifestyle tips on nutrition and sleep, this guide covers a comprehensive range of topics to support your physical and emotional well-being.

As you turn each page, you'll find exercises and a new perspective on what your body can achieve, regardless of age. The potential outcomes—increased strength, better balance, and enhanced flexibility—are just the beginning. Embrace this journey with an open mind. Let every seated movement bring you one step closer to a more active and independent life.

I am with you on this journey. Together, let's move towards a healthier, more vibrant future. Here's to finding strength, balance, and joy in every seat.

CHAPTER ONE

UNDERSTANDING CHAIR EXERCISES

Have you ever paused to reflect on the simple joy of movement? Many of us have experienced physical limitations that put our favorite activities out of reach. This chapter is about rediscovering those possibilities through chair exercises, a form of physical activity designed to accommodate and enhance your mobility, regardless of your current fitness level.

Chair exercises are a beacon of hope for many who face challenges with conventional exercise routines due to age, injury, or disability. These exercises provide a safe, flexible, and incredibly effective way to improve your health and regain independence. Let's explore how this exercise can become vital to your daily life, bringing you closer to a more active and fulfilled lifestyle.

1.1 WHAT ARE CHAIR EXERCISES? DEFINING YOUR PATH TO MOBILITY

Chair exercises are adaptive physical activities you can perform while seated, making them an ideal choice if standing workouts are uncomfortable or unfeasible. These exercises encompass a broad spectrum of movements designed to enhance cardiovascular health, muscle strength, flexibility, and balance. The beauty of chair exercises lies in their low-impact nature, which significantly reduces the stress on your joints while still providing the physical benefits of exercise.

Versatility of Chair Exercises

One of the most significant advantages of chair exercises is their versatility. Whether you aim to improve heart health with light cardio, strengthen muscles through resistance training, or enhance flexibility and balance with yoga-inspired stretches, a chair exercise meets your needs. This versatility helps maintain a comprehensive fitness routine and keeps the workouts exciting and engaging. You can tailor your sessions to focus more on areas you need to improve, such as strengthening your legs to make climbing stairs easier. Alternatively, focus on your upper body and core muscles to ensure you can carry groceries or efficiently perform other daily tasks.

Accessibility of Chair Exercises

Integrating chair exercises into your daily routine is surprisingly easy. You don't need specialized equipment or ample space; you need a stable chair and the willingness to move. This accessibility makes it possible to exercise in the comfort of your own home, regardless of the weather or time of day. It's an empowering way to independently maintain your fitness routine, ensuring you can work out safely and comfortably without expensive gym memberships or equipment.

Adaptability of Chair Exercises

Another appeal of chair exercises is their adaptability. Suppose you're just starting or have significant mobility limitations. In that case, you can perform gentle movements that gradually build strength and flexibility. As your fitness improves, you can increase the intensity of your workouts by incorporating weights, resistance bands, or more complex movements—all from your chair. This adaptability helps you continuously challenge your body in new ways. It allows you to customize exercises to suit your health conditions and physical capabilities.

For those needing additional motivation or guidance, consider integrating a visual element like a chart of daily exercises. This could include a simple checklist or photos illustrating each movement. Having a visual reference not only aids in ensuring you perform each exercise correctly but also helps track your progress, keeping you motivated and engaged in your fitness journey.

1.2 THE TOP 5 BENEFITS OF CHAIR EXERCISES FOR SENIORS

Engaging in regular chair exercises provides a plethora of health benefits that extend far beyond simple physical fitness. For many seniors, the motivation to start might stem from the desire to improve mobility and flexibility. As we age, our joints often show signs of wear; they stiffen and ache, making daily movements more challenging. Regular chair exercises allow these joints to move through their full range of motion, effectively lubricating them like oiling a squeaky hinge. This movement reduces stiffness and alleviates pain associated with conditions such as arthritis. Imagine bending to tie your shoelaces or reaching up to grab a can from the top shelf without a twinge of pain—this can be a reality with consistent practice. Flexibility is crucial, not just for performing everyday tasks but also for preventing injuries that can occur from sudden movements.

Strengthening muscles and bones is another critical benefit that cannot be overstated. As the body ages, it naturally loses muscle mass and bone density, a condition exacerbated by inactivity. The chair exercises that involve resistance, like lifting small weights or pulling against resistance bands, encourage muscle growth and bone fortification. This kind of training signals your body to bone up, quite literally, thereby reducing the risk of osteoporosis. More robust muscles support your joints better and decrease the burden on your bones, which can be particularly beneficial for those with joint issues. Each time you lift a weight or pull against a band, you're not just working on your muscles; you're building a sturdier, more resilient frame that can withstand the test of time.

Balance and stability are among the most crucial factors in preventing falls, a common concern for many seniors. Chair exercises that strengthen the core and other stabilizing muscles are invaluable. These exercises teach your body to maintain its center of gravity, improving your ability to react to shifts in balance and reducing the likelihood of falls. This aspect of chair exercises is about giving you the confidence to move freely, knowing your body has the strength and stability to support itself. Whether navigating a crowded room or standing up from a chair, improved balance means a significantly lower fall risk, enhancing overall independence.

The mental health benefits of regular exercise are well-documented and vast. Engaging in chair exercises can lead to reductions in stress, anxiety, and depression. Physical activity triggers the release of endorphins, often called feel-good hormones, which can create feelings of euphoria and general well-being. It's not just about the biochemical changes; however, completing a workout can boost self-esteem and accomplishment, combatting feelings of isolation or depression that sometimes accompany aging. Imagine starting your day with movements that awaken your body, clear your mind, and elevate your mood. This mental clarity and positivity can carry over into every part of your day.

Lastly, the social benefits of chair exercises can be significant, mainly in a group setting. Whether it's a class at a local community center or a regular meet-up with a friend or family member to go through a routine, these interactions contribute to a sense of community and belonging. They provide a forum for encouragement and motivation, emotional support, and companionship. Even those who prefer to exercise from the comfort of home can engage with others through online platforms where many chair exercise programs are shared. This sense of connection is vital, as social engagement has improved longevity and quality of life.

Each of these benefits feeds into the next, holistically enhancing your overall well-being. Regular chair exercises can transform how you feel physically and mentally, enrich your social life, and provide you with the tools to maintain and enhance your independence. As we continue to explore the impact of these exercises, remember that each movement is a step towards a healthier, more vibrant you.

1.3 SAFETY FIRST: PREPARING YOUR SPACE AND CHOOSING THE RIGHT CHAIR

When you incorporate chair exercises into your routine, the first step is ensuring your environment is optimized for safety and comfort. This preparation is not just about the physical space but also involves selecting the right equipment and consulting with professionals to tailor the exercises to your needs. Let's explore how you can set up your space, choose the appropriate chair, dress correctly, and seek medical advice to maximize the benefits of your workouts while minimizing any risks.

Space Preparation

A well-organized space is fundamental to a safe and effective workout. You'll need an area free of clutter that provides enough room to perform movements fully and freely. Your exercise space should allow you to extend your arms and legs without touching furniture or walls. This could include moving some items aside if you're exercising in a living room or a bedroom. Ensure the floor area is clean and dry to prevent slips; using a non-slip mat can provide additional stability if you're on a hard surface. Good lighting is crucial to ensure you can see what you are doing and avoid any potential hazards that might not be obvious in dim light. Remember, the goal is to create a haven that invites daily movement without concerns about obstacles.

Selecting the Right Chair

The choice of chair is critical in chair exercises. An ideal chair is sturdy and stable without wheels, as rolling chairs can shift unexpectedly and lead to falls. The chair should also be without arms to allow freedom of movement during exercises. The chair's height is another important consideration; when sitting, your feet should rest flat on the floor, and your thighs should be parallel to the ground. This position helps maintain proper posture and balance during exercises. Testing the chair before starting your exercises is a good practice—ensure it feels solid and comfortable as you sit and stand from it repeatedly.

Wearing Appropriate Clothing and Footwear

What you wear during your exercises can significantly impact your safety and effectiveness. Choose comfortable clothes and give you a full range of motion. Fabrics that stretch and breathe are preferable, as they accommodate movement and reduce the risk of overheating. Footwear is equally important; while it might be tempting to go barefoot or wear slippers, sturdy shoes with non-slip soles are safest. They provide the necessary support and grip, helping prevent slips and falls during your workout. Ensure these shoes fit correctly —neither tight nor loose—as improper footwear can lead to blisters, calluses, and other foot ailments that could sideline your exercise goals.

Consulting Healthcare Providers

Before starting any new exercise regimen, particularly if you have pre-existing health conditions or concerns, it's wise to consult with a healthcare provider. This step is crucial, as it helps ensure that the exercises you plan to do are safe and beneficial for your specific health situation. Your doctor can advise which exercises to avoid and which might be particularly helpful. They might also recommend a session with a physical therapist who can tailor an exercise program to fit your needs safely. This personalized approach not only maximizes the effectiveness of your workouts but also minimizes the risk of injury, ensuring that your path to increased mobility and improved health is as smooth and safe as possible.

As we move forward, remember that the foundation of any successful exercise program is safety. By preparing your space, selecting the right equipment, wearing appropriate clothing, and consulting with professionals, you are setting yourself up for success. While seemingly simple, these steps are vital in creating a workout environment that supports your health and well-being, allowing you to reap the full benefits of chair exercises without undue risk. Here's to moving confidently and safely towards a healthier you.

CHAPTER TWO
OVERCOMING COMMON BARRIERS

A s we age, our bodies often present us with fresh challenges, and embracing an active lifestyle can sometimes feel like an uphill battle. However, the beauty of chair exercises lies in their adaptability, making them a valuable tool for overcoming these physical barriers. This chapter is dedicated to helping you navigate some of the common hurdles you might face, mainly focusing on limited mobility, which should not deter your aspirations for a fitter and more vibrant life.

2.1 NAVIGATING LIMITED MOBILITY: EXERCISES TAILORED FOR ALL ABILITIES

Understanding the diverse range of mobility levels among seniors is crucial in appreciating how adaptable chair exercises can be. Mobility challenges can vary widely from one individual to another, influenced by factors such as age, medical conditions, or the aftermath of surgery. Recognizing this diversity is the first step in creating a workout routine that respects your body's current state while gently encouraging its potential. Chair exercises can be finely tuned to meet you exactly where you are in your physical capabilities.

Customizing Exercises: Strategies for Tailoring Exercises to Individual Capabilities

Every individual's body has its own set of strengths and limitations, and acknowledging this is key to a successful exercise regimen. Chair exercises are wonderfully versatile and can be modified to cater to your specific needs. For instance, if standing poses are too challenging, they can be performed while seated, ensuring you still engage the same muscle groups but in a manageable and safe manner. On days when you feel more agile, incorporating standing variations next to a chair for support can help build confidence and balance.

For those who find specific movements too strenuous, introducing props such as resistance bands, soft balls, or light weights can make a significant difference. These tools not only aid in making exercises more accessible but also add a layer of challenge that can be adjusted according to your comfort and progress. For example, a resistance band can help perform an arm lift by providing support and reducing the strain on your muscles and joints. This adaptability ensures that your body is always engaged at just the right level of challenge.

Using Props and Assistive Devices

Incorporating props and assistive devices can significantly enhance the effectiveness of your exercises while ensuring safety and comfort. Resistance bands are excellent for building strength without heavy weights, making them perfect for muscle toning and improving flexibility. Soft balls can be used to enhance grip strength and coordination, while light dumbbells can help build muscle mass gradually. Each of these tools can be used to modify exercises to your comfort level, allowing for a gradual increase in difficulty as your strength and confidence grow.

Encouragement and Realistic Expectations: Fostering a Positive Mindset

Setting realistic goals and maintaining a positive mindset are as important as the exercises. It's essential to acknowledge and celebrate every little progress, no matter how small it may seem. Every movement counts towards a larger goal of greater mobility and improved health. Setting achievable milestones and recognizing your achievements provides a significant psychological boost. It helps build a positive association with exercise, transforming it from a daunting task into an enjoyable and rewarding activity. Celebrate the days when you can stretch a little further or hold a pose a bit longer; each is a stepping stone to greater independence and health.

Chair exercises offer a flexible and effective way for seniors to enhance their physical health, irrespective of their mobility levels. By understanding and embracing their adaptability, you can create a personalized exercise routine that respects your body's current capabilities while gently pushing its boundaries. This approach ensures safety and makes staying active enjoyable and fulfilling, paving the way for a healthier, more independent life.

2.2 EASING FEARS: INJURY PREVENTION THROUGH PROPER TECHNIQUE

One of the most common concerns you might have when starting a new exercise program, especially as a senior, is the risk of injury. This is a valid concern, as our bodies become more susceptible to strains and other injuries as we age. However, focusing on proper technique and form can significantly reduce this risk and make your exercise routine safe and beneficial. Maintaining correct posture and movements during your exercises is crucial. It ensures that each body part is aligned correctly, minimizing undue stress on any joint or muscle group. For instance, when doing a seated leg extension, it's essential to sit upright, engage your core, and extend your leg smoothly without jerking. This helps effectively work the targeted muscles and prevents strain on the knee joint and surrounding muscles.

Starting slowly with low-intensity exercises is another critical strategy in injury prevention. It's tempting to dive into more challenging routines to see quick results. Still, gradual progression is safer and more effective in the long run. Begin with exercises that you find manageable, and gradually increase the intensity as your body adapts. This approach strengthens your muscles and joints over time, building a solid foundation to handle more strenuous activities without injury. For example, suppose you're new to chair exercises. Start with simple seated stretches and gradually incorporate light weights or resistance bands as your flexibility and strength improve.

Recognizing the signs of overexertion is also essential for maintaining a safe exercise routine. It's important to listen to your body and understand the difference between pushing yourself healthily and too hard. Symptoms of overexertion can include excessive fatigue, dizziness, breathlessness, and pain. If you experience any of these symptoms, pausing and rest is crucial. Pushing through pain or discomfort can lead to severe injuries. It's better to stop and consult a healthcare provider if these symptoms persist. Understanding your body's limits and permitting yourself to rest when needed is not a setback—it's a smart strategy for long-term fitness and health.

Lastly, seeking professional guidance can significantly affect how safely and effectively you perform your exercises. Consulting with a physical therapist who understands the unique needs of seniors can provide you with a personalized exercise plan that accounts for any specific health concerns or mobility limitations you have. Additionally, exercise videos designed for seniors can help you visualize the correct forms and techniques. These resources often include modifications for various exercises, ensuring you can adapt them to your current fitness level. Whether through professional consultations or carefully selected instructional videos, getting expert advice can help you exercise confidently and safely, making your fitness routine a rewarding part of your daily life.

By focusing on proper technique, starting slow, recognizing signs of overexertion, and seeking professional guidance, you can enjoy the myriad benefits of chair exercises without fear of injury. This thoughtful exercise approach helps prevent injuries and enriches your experience, making it more enjoyable and sustainable in the long run. Remember, the goal is to enhance your health and well-being, and taking these precautions ensures you can continue doing so safely and effectively.

2.3 MAKING EXERCISE ACCESSIBLE: SOLUTIONS FOR VISION AND SPACE LIMITATIONS

For many seniors, particularly those with visual impairments or living in smaller spaces, starting an exercise routine might seem fraught with obstacles. However, with a few thoughtful adaptations, chair exercises can become a highly accessible and enjoyable part of your daily routine, ensuring you remain active and healthy regardless of these challenges.

Adapting Exercises for Visual Impairments

Traditional visual cues in exercise routines are only sometimes effective for those with limited vision. However, auditory cues can be an excellent alternative, guiding you through workouts with clear, descriptive instructions. Consider audio exercise programs designed specifically for visually impaired individuals, which detail each movement step-by-step, allowing you to perform each exercise safely and effectively. Additionally, textured mats can be helpful by providing tactile cues through different surface textures, helping you orient yourself in the space and maintain balance.

Moreover, engaging more actively with instructors or workout companions who can provide verbal cues during exercises can enhance your workout experience. This can be through live in-person or online classes, where instructors give real-time feedback and directions. Alternatively, you can work out alongside a friend or family member who can describe the movements and offer immediate assistance if needed.

Maximizing Small Spaces

Living in a compact space doesn't mean you have to compromise on your exercise routine. Chair exercises are particularly suited for small environments requiring very little room. To make the most out of your available space, consider rearranging furniture to create a temporary workout area. Even a tiny cleared area can provide sufficient space for a wide range of seated exercises.

Suppose you're concerned about maintaining a permanent setup. In that case, lightweight chairs can be easily moved before and after workouts, ensuring your living area remains functional for other activities throughout the day. Additionally, using foldable or multi-functional furniture can allow you to quickly adapt your living space for exercise and then return it to its usual setup with minimal effort.

Utilizing Household Items

Innovative use of household items can also make chair exercises more engaging and effective without requiring specialized equipment. Everyday items such as filled water bottles can double as weights, and socks can be used on hardwood floors to perform seated leg slides, which can help strengthen your leg muscles. A sturdy wall or the back of a heavy couch can support stretching exercises.

These simple substitutions make it easier to start exercising without additional expenses and help keep your routine varied and exciting. This approach encourages creativity in your workouts, making the exercise experience fun and beneficial.

Overcoming Isolation

For seniors with social isolation, engaging in exercise can sometimes feel like a solitary endeavor. However, numerous resources can help you connect with others and add a social element to your workouts. Online exercise classes offer a way to participate in guided workouts from home while interacting with instructors and fellow participants through live video sessions. Additionally, many fitness programs on DVDs or television are designed with seniors in mind, providing routines you can follow along with others and fostering a sense of community.

Local community centers often offer chair exercise classes, which can be a great way to meet people and stay active. Even if you prefer to exercise at home, scheduling regular workout times with friends over a video call can give you a similar social experience. These interactions not only make exercising more enjoyable but also help build a support network, keeping you motivated and engaged.

By adapting exercises to accommodate visual impairments, making the most of small spaces, utilizing everyday items for workouts, and finding ways to overcome social isolation, chair exercises can be a highly accessible and enjoyable way to maintain your health and wellness. These adaptations ensure you can stay active and engaged, regardless of physical or environmental limitations.

As this chapter concludes, remember that each adaptation enhances your ability to exercise effectively and contributes to a broader sense of independence and well-being. The strategies discussed here pave the way for a more inclusive approach to fitness, ensuring that everyone can enjoy the benefits of physical activity regardless of their circumstances. As we move forward, we'll explore how to further enhance your exercise routine by integrating strength and muscle toning exercises, ensuring a comprehensive approach to your fitness journey.

CHAPTER THREE
SETTING UP FOR SUCCESS

I magine stepping into a space uniquely yours, tailored for comfort, safety, and effectiveness in your pursuit of health through chair exercises. Setting up for success in your exercise routine is about something other than having the most expensive equipment or a professional gym setup. Instead, it's about creating a safe, comfortable environment that encourages regular practice. This chapter is dedicated to helping you assemble the right toolkit that supports your fitness journey without cluttering your space or complicating your routines.

3.1 EQUIPMENT ESSENTIALS: SIMPLIFYING YOUR EXERCISE TOOLKIT

When starting with chair exercises, the beauty lies in the simplicity of the equipment needed. At its core, all you need is a stable chair and comfortable clothing that allows unrestricted movement. The right chair—sturdy, without arms, and at a height where your feet rest flat when seated—becomes your foundation. This isn't just any chair; it's your partner in the quest for improved health. It supports your body as you perform exercises that enhance strength, flexibility, and balance.

Minimalist Approach

Adopting a minimalist approach to your exercise equipment is economical. It clears your space and mind for a focused workout session. You don't need expensive or bulky equipment to achieve your fitness goals. A simple setup encourages you to maintain regular workouts. Also, it makes it easier to keep your exercise area tidy and inviting. Remember, the less hassle it is to start your workout, the more likely you will stick with your routine. Comfortable, breathable clothing and sound, supportive shoes complete your essential toolkit. These items you likely already own make a difference in your workout experience by providing comfort and preventing injuries.

Optional Equipment

While the basics are often sufficient, incorporating a few optional items can enhance your workout and provide variety. Resistance bands, for example, are a fantastic addition to your toolkit. They're affordable, versatile, and can be stored easily without taking up much space. Light dumbbells or even a couple of water bottles can serve as weights to add a little resistance to your exercises, helping to build muscle strength more effectively. A non-slip mat can also be beneficial, especially if you have hardwood or tile floors, providing a stable surface to prevent slips during standing or seated exercises.

Investment vs. DIY

Whether to invest in quality exercise equipment or use DIY alternatives comes down to a balance of cost, effectiveness, and safety. While DIY options can be cost-effective and are a good start, investing in professionally designed equipment for exercise can offer better durability and safety. For instance, professional resistance bands are designed to withstand high stress and usage, reducing the risk of snapping and injury. However, if budgets are tight, starting with household items like towels (for resistance) or a sturdy chair can also support your initial steps into chair exercises.

Safety Checks

Regularly checking your equipment for signs of wear and tear is crucial in ensuring your safety during workouts. Inspect items like resistance bands and dumbbells for any damage before use. Check your chair for stability, and ensure your exercise mat remains non-slip. Keeping your equipment in good condition prevents injuries and reinforces your commitment to an active lifestyle. Set a regular schedule, perhaps at the beginning of each month, to inspect your exercise equipment. This routine ensures safety, allows you to reflect on your progress, and renews your dedication to your fitness goals.

Setting up for success in chair exercises doesn't require a significant investment or a lot of space. With a few simple tools and regular safety checks, you can create a safe, effective environment for your workouts. This setup process is integral to your fitness journey, preparing you physically, mentally, and emotionally for the health improvements ahead. As you move forward, remember that each piece of your toolkit supports your path to greater mobility, strength, and independence, making each exercise session a step toward a healthier you.

3.2 PERSONALIZING YOUR ROUTINE: LISTENING TO YOUR BODY'S NEEDS

Creating a fitness routine that resonates with your needs is not just about following a set of exercises; it's about understanding and responding to your body's unique responses and requirements. This personalized approach ensures that your activities boost your health and bring you joy and satisfaction, keeping you motivated and engaged over time. It begins with setting personalized fitness goals aligned with your health, mobility, and interests.

When considering your goals, consider what you wish to achieve through your chair exercises. You may want to improve your flexibility enough to play with your grandchildren without discomfort, or you may aim to build enough endurance to enjoy walks in the park. It could be as simple as enhancing your balance to feel more confident moving around your home. Whatever your aspirations, let them guide your exercise plan. This alignment ensures that your routine remains relevant and exciting, crucial for long-term adherence. Reflect on activities you used to enjoy or new ones you wish to explore and consider how improving your physical health could help you engage more fully with those interests.

Listening to your body's cues during exercise is another vital component of personalizing your routine. Your body communicates through signals such as breathlessness, muscle fatigue, or even the exhilarating rush of energy after a good workout. Learning to interpret these signs can help you adjust your exercise intensity, duration, and form to optimize your workouts without risking discomfort or injury. For instance, if you notice undue strain in your joints during a particular movement, consider modifying that exercise to reduce the impact or consulting a physical therapist for alternative exercises that achieve similar results without discomfort. Similarly, on days when you feel vibrant and strong, you might slightly increase the intensity of your workout to push your limits gently. This responsiveness keeps your routine safe and dynamically aligned with your changing fitness levels and health status.

Incorporating a variety of exercises into your routine is crucial not just for physical health but also for mental engagement. Engaging different muscle groups helps achieve a balanced improvement in muscle strength, flexibility, and cardiovascular health. Additionally, variety keeps the routine exciting and fun, essential in maintaining long-term motivation. You might include a mix of strength training, flexibility stretches, and light cardiovascular exercises like chair marching or seated dance routines. Each exercise type brings benefits and challenges, ensuring your body constantly adapts and improves. Furthermore, varying your activities can help prevent the kind of overuse injuries that occur from repeating the same movements too frequently.

Finally, adjusting your exercise routine in response to fluctuations in energy levels and health status is a practical aspect of personalization. On days when you feel full of vigor, you might extend your exercise time or include a few more challenging exercises. Conversely, when you feel low in energy or are recovering from a minor illness, it's wise to scale back your activities to match what your body can handle comfortably. This flexibility in your approach prevents physical strain and respects your body's natural rhythms and needs, promoting a healthier, more supportive relationship with your exercise regimen.

By setting personal goals, listening to your body's cues, incorporating various exercises, and adjusting to daily fluctuations in energy and health, you create a fitness routine that aligns with your life. This personalized approach enhances the effectiveness of your workouts. It ensures that your exercise routine is a joyous and integral part of your everyday life, tailored just for you.

3.3 STAYING MOTIVATED: SETTING REALISTIC GOALS AND TRACKING PROGRESS

One of the foundational elements of sustained exercise commitment is the ability to set and reach achievable goals. This process isn't just about aiming for objectives and crafting milestones well-matched to your current skills and aspirations. Setting realistic goals does not mean they can't be challenging; instead, it ensures that they are attainable within a reasonable timeframe and with available resources, thereby preventing feelings of frustration and discouragement. For instance, if improving balance is your goal, a realistic milestone could be to perform a balance exercise without support for 10 seconds. Once this goal is comfortably met, you can extend the time or add complexity, like closing your eyes while balancing.

Tracking your progress is equally critical as it provides tangible evidence of your improvements, no matter how small. This can be incredibly motivating and can be done in various ways. A simple method is keeping an exercise journal where you note the type of exercises performed, the duration, and how you felt during and after the sessions. This record tracks your progress and helps identify patterns that might affect your performance, such as better energy levels at certain times of the day. Fitness apps can be an excellent tool for those comfortable with technology. Many apps are designed to record physical activities automatically, summarize your weekly or monthly progress, and even offer virtual badges or rewards as you meet your goals.

Celebrating successes plays a crucial role in maintaining your exercise momentum. Every milestone reached should be acknowledged and celebrated, whether treating yourself to a new book, enjoying a special meal, or simply sharing your achievements with friends or family. These celebrations reinforce positive feelings associated with your fitness achievements and can be powerful motivators to keep progressing. For example, completing a month-long daily exercise streak might be celebrated by purchasing a new piece of workout clothing or equipment, symbolizing both a reward and an investment in your continuing fitness journey.

Lastly, the support of others can significantly enhance your motivational levels. Engaging with a network of family, friends, or an online community who share your commitment to maintaining an active lifestyle can provide encouragement, share valuable tips, and even offer gentle accountability. Having an exercise buddy or joining an in-person or online group helps maintain a regular exercise schedule. Moreover, sharing your experiences and challenges with others who understand and support your goals can transform the sometimes-monotonous act of daily exercise into a social, enjoyable, and gratifying endeavor.

In essence, the journey to maintaining an active lifestyle through chair exercises is greatly supported by setting achievable goals, tracking your progress through convenient methods, celebrating every success, and engaging with supportive networks. These elements foster sustained motivation and enrich your exercise experience, making it a rewarding and integral part of your life.

As we wrap up this chapter on setting up for success, remember that the tools, personal adjustments, and motivational strategies you've learned here are not just about facilitating physical activity —they're about crafting a lifestyle that embraces and sustains physical wellness. With your toolkit ready, your routines personalized, and your motivation securely anchored, you're well on your way to reaping the full benefits of your exercise regimen. In the next chapter, we'll delve into the specifics of enhancing strength and muscle tone, building on the foundation you've established to optimize your physical health outcomes further.

CHAPTER FOUR

ENHANCING STRENGTH AND MUSCLE TONE

S trength isn't just the ability to lift heavy objects; it's the foundation that supports your body's overall function and mobility. As we age, maintaining muscle tone and strength becomes crucial for carrying out daily activities and ensuring a resilient and healthy body. This chapter is dedicated to enhancing your upper body strength by using one of the most versatile pieces of equipment available for chair exercises: resistance bands. These tools are not merely accessories but allies in your quest to maintain and build strength in a way that respects your body's capabilities and needs.

4.1 ARM STRENGTH: USING RESISTANCE BANDS FOR TONING

Equipment Introduction

Resistance bands come in various types, each suited to different fitness levels and exercise routines. These bands typically range in resistance from very light, suitable for beginners or those with significant mobility limitations, to very heavy, for those looking to challenge their muscle strength seriously. The most common types include flat therapy bands, often used in physical therapy, and tubular bands, which may come with handles and offer more resistance. You can incorporate each type into your exercise routine to help tone and strengthen your arms, shoulders, and upper back.

For seniors, starting with lighter, flat bands is advisable as they are easier to handle and less intimidating. With these bands, you can stretch and strengthen muscles with a minimal risk of injury. As you are comfortable with the exercises and your muscle strength improves, you may progress to tubular bands with handles, which can provide a more significant challenge and help further enhance muscle tone.

Exercise Variety

Using resistance bands or dumbbells for arm toning provides a range of exercises that target different muscle groups in the upper body. Here are some practical exercises to incorporate into your routine:

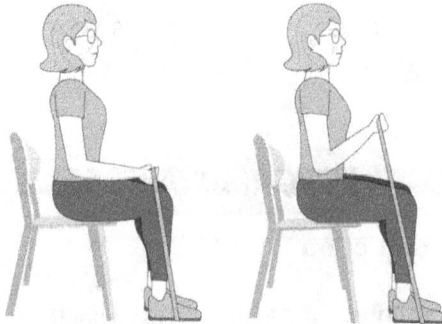

Seated Bicep Curls: Sit upright on your chair with your feet flat on the floor. Hold the ends of the resistance band under your feet and grasp the other ends in your hands. Slowly curl your hands up towards your shoulders, keeping your elbows close to your body. Then, slowly release back down. This exercise targets the biceps in the front of your upper arms. Dumbbells can also be used.

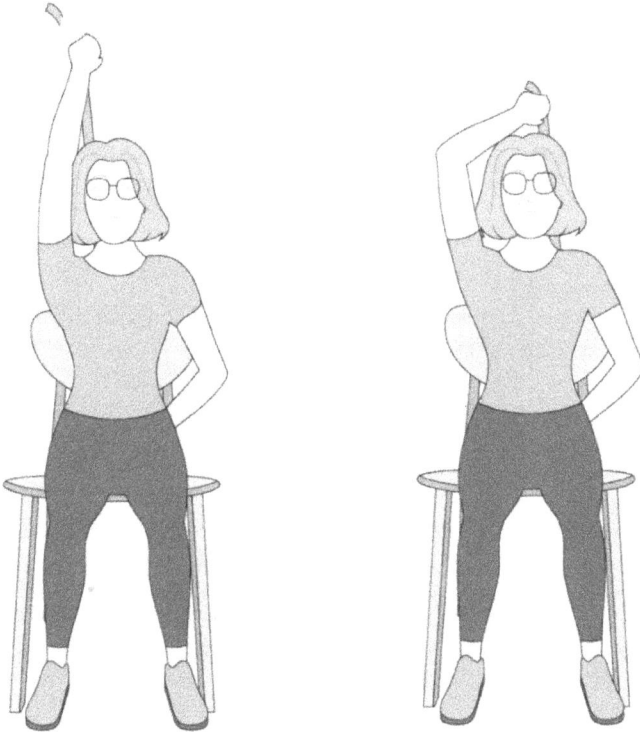

Seated Tricep Extensions: Start with one end of the band held in hand and raised above your head and the other secured by your opposite hand behind your back. Extend the upper arm to straighten it above your head, then slowly bring it back to the bent position. This focuses on the tricep muscles at the back of your upper arms.

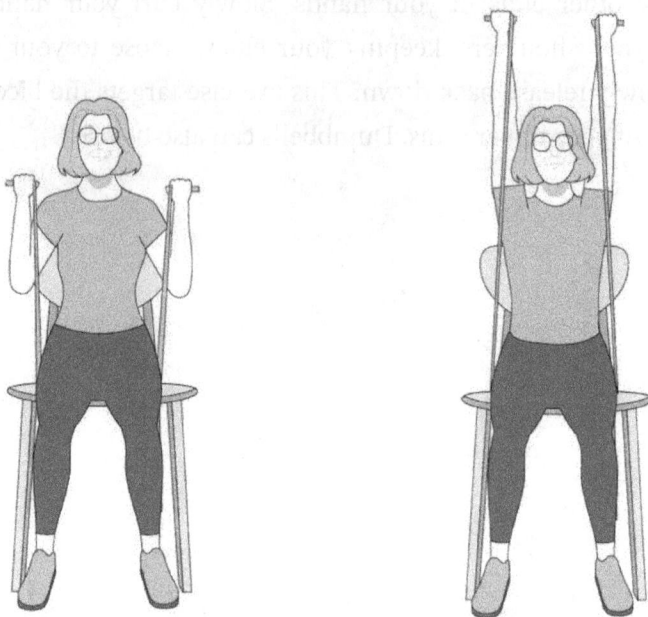

Seated Shoulder Press: With a resistance band lay the band centered across the front edge of the chair. Sitting upright at the edge of the chair on top of the band with feet flat and spread shoulder width apart. Take ahold of the band ends and place your arms in a goalpost shape. Your triceps should be parallel with the floor and at shoulder height. Then press your arms straight up and slightly to the front so that you can just see them. If they go behind your head there is risk for a neck strain.

Seated Side Extension: Sit upright at the edge of the chair with feet flat and spread shoulder width apart. This can be performed using dumbbells or resistance bands. With bands lay the band across the floor spread equally under the front chair legs. Then holding both ends of the band pull arms straight upward to shoulder height.

With dumbbells, have one in each hand hanging along your side and raise upward from the sides to shoulder height.

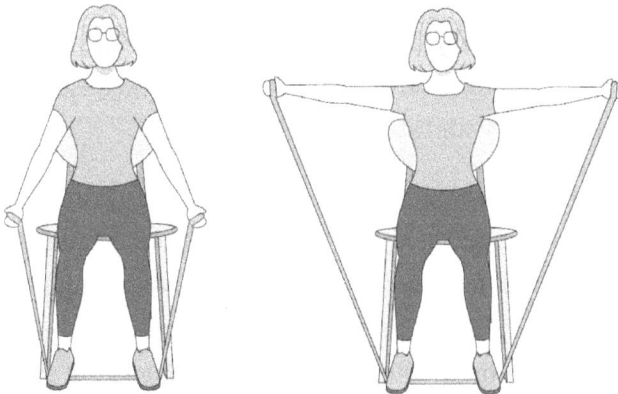

Performing these exercises regularly can significantly improve arm strength and flexibility, contributing to better functionality in daily tasks such as lifting or carrying groceries.

Safety Precautions

While resistance bands are relatively safe, proper form and technique are crucial to avoid injury. Ensure the band is securely anchored under your feet or other stable object when performing exercises to prevent it from snapping back. Start each exercise slowly to familiarize yourself with the movement, ensuring your body is aligned correctly to avoid unnecessary strain. If you experience pain beyond normal muscle fatigue, stop the exercise and consult a professional to ensure you're performing it correctly.

Progress and Adaptation

As your strength improves, it's important to continue challenging your muscles to enhance muscle tone and functionality further. One way to do this is by increasing the resistance of the bands you use. Progressing from lighter to heavier bands can help maintain the challenge as your strength improves. Additionally, you can increase the number of repetitions or sets of exercises to continue building endurance and strength.

Regularly incorporating these exercises into your routine can improve your upper body strength, making everyday activities easier and reducing the risk of falls and other injuries. As you enhance your arm strength, you'll see improvements in your physical capabilities, confidence, and overall quality of life. Remember, each stretch and curl is a step toward a stronger, more capable you.

4.2 CORE STABILITY: SAFE EXERCISES TO STRENGTHEN YOUR ABDOMINALS

The core of your body is like the foundation of a house; it supports everything else above and around it. When your core is strong, it supports your spine and upper body. It enhances balance and stability, making everyday activities more accessible and safer. Strengthening your core can significantly improve your posture, reduce back pain, and enhance overall mobility. This is why core exercises are integral to any fitness regimen, especially for seniors more susceptible to falls and back injuries.

Core strength exercises are not just about sculpting a toned belly; they are crucial for maintaining functional fitness and independence. Regularly engaging your core muscles helps safeguard your lower back from undue strain during movements like bending or twisting. For seniors, this can mean fewer injuries and less pain, contributing to a better quality of life and greater autonomy. Therefore, engaging in exercises that specifically target these muscles is not just about fitness but about fostering a body that efficiently supports your active lifestyle.

Practical abdominal exercises can be performed right from your chair, making them safe and convenient. A simple yet effective exercise to start with is the seated march.

Seated Bicycle Crunch: While sitting upright at the forward edge and both feet flat on the surface, lean back slightly and bring your hands behind your head. Bring one foot off the floor and toward the middle your chest. Engage your core and bring your opposite elbow to your knee. Relax and gradually return to your starting position. Repeat with the other side. If this is to hard at the beginning then just perform using your torso and keep your feet firmly planted until you are confident enough to raise your knees.

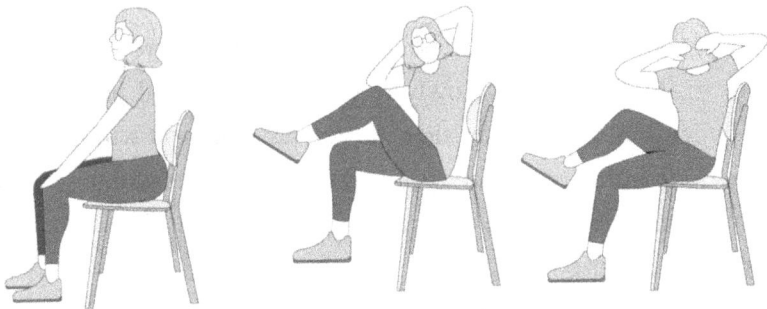

Seated Twist: Hold your arms in front of you with elbows bent, and slowly twist your torso to one side, then the other. This movement engages the deeper abdominal muscles and helps improve your rotational flexibility, essential for tasks like looking behind you or reaching for objects on the side.

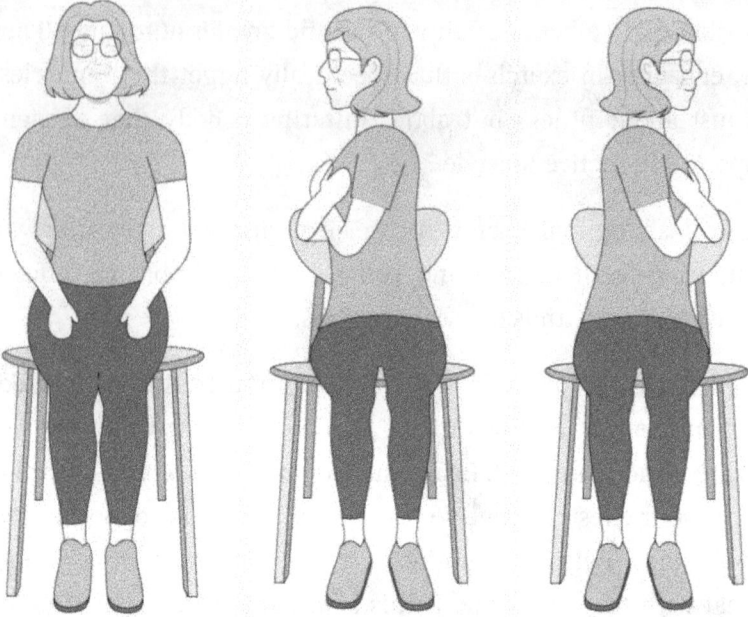

<u>Seated Side Bend</u>: While sitting upright with back straight and both feet flat on the surface, you allow both arms to hang straight down. Then you slowly bend to one side at your waist as your hand gets closer to the floor. Then slowly return to the neutral position and slowly bending to the other side. As you advance you will get closer to the floor and may consider using dumbbells. This will target your oblique muscles. Your lateral flexibility will improve thus promoting better posture.

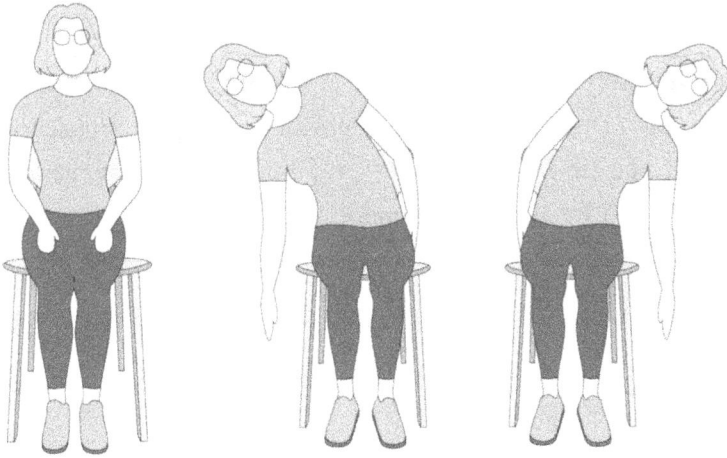

<u>Seated Knee Tucks</u>: Sitting upright and with core engaged, bring your knees as close to your chest as you are able. Then bring them back down and tap the floor. You can use the edge of the chair to hold as support, once you've mastered this exercise you can hold your arms straight outward and tucking your knees between. This exercise with help strengthen your lower abdominal muscles.

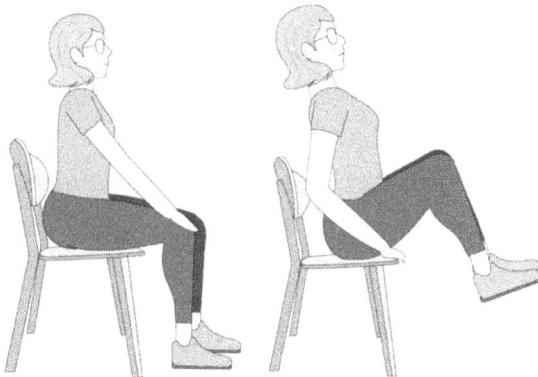

Breathing correctly during these exercises enhances their effectiveness and ensures you properly engage your core muscles. The technique involves breathing deeply and exhaling forcefully when you exert the most effort. For instance, in the seated twist, you would inhale as you prepare to twist and exhale as you perform the twist. This type of breathing helps activate your core muscles and prevents you from holding your breath, which can increase blood pressure. Proper core engagement is achieved by imagining you pulling your belly button towards your spine. This action helps stabilize your torso and protects your spine during exercises.

Incorporating these core-strengthening exercises into your overall chair exercise routine should be done thoughtfully to ensure a balanced development of your body's capabilities. It's beneficial to begin your workout session with a few core exercises as they warm up the muscles that stabilize your spine, preparing your body for other exercises. Alternatively, you can intersperse core exercises between exercises targeting different areas, keeping your core engaged and active throughout the session. This approach maintains a balanced workout and keeps your energy levels distributed evenly throughout the exercise routine, helping to prevent fatigue.

By consistently integrating core exercises into your daily routine, you lay a strong foundation for improved health and mobility. These exercises, while simple, play a crucial role in enhancing your physical stability and reducing the risk of falls and injuries. As you continue to strengthen your core, you'll likely notice improvements in your ability to perform daily tasks with greater ease and confidence, making your everyday life safer and more enjoyable.

4.3 LEG AND GLUTE WORKOUTS: BUILDING LOWER BODY STRENGTH

Strengthening the legs and glutes is pivotal for maintaining balance and mobility and performing everyday activities with ease and confidence. Seated leg and glute exercises provide a safe, effective way to build strength in these crucial muscle groups without needing standing or heavy equipment. These exercises are particularly beneficial as they help maintain muscle mass and bone density, which can diminish as we age.

Seated Leg Lift: While sitting upright at the edge of the chair, extend one leg straight and lift it to a challenging yet manageable height; hold it momentarily, then slowly lower it back down. Repeating this exercise, alternating legs, helps build muscle symmetry and strength throughout the lower body. This movement targets the thigh muscles and engages the glutes, especially as you resist gravity on the way down. You can use the edge of the chair to hold as support, once you've mastered this exercise you can hold your arms straight out to the sides. This is a foundational exercise that significantly benefits the lower body.

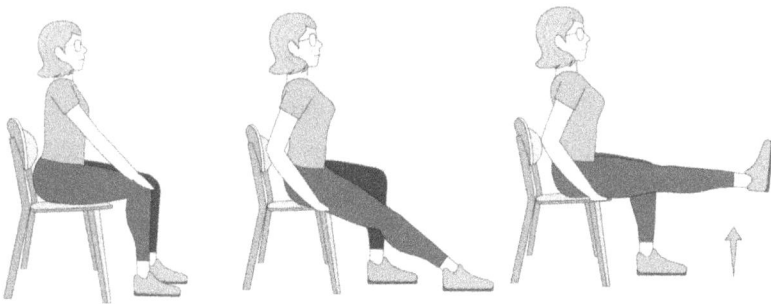

Seated Chair Squats: Some refer to this exercises as Sit-to-Stands. Sit upright at the edge of the chair with feet shoulder width apart and toes angled slightly outward, engage your core and chest sticking out; keep your hands out in front of you for balance. Then slowly begin to sit up until completely standing, keeping your knees apart. Utilizing your hips to generate the momentum rather than using your knees. Squeeze your buttocks/glutes together to engage the muscles for additional muscles toning. Then sit back down and repeat.

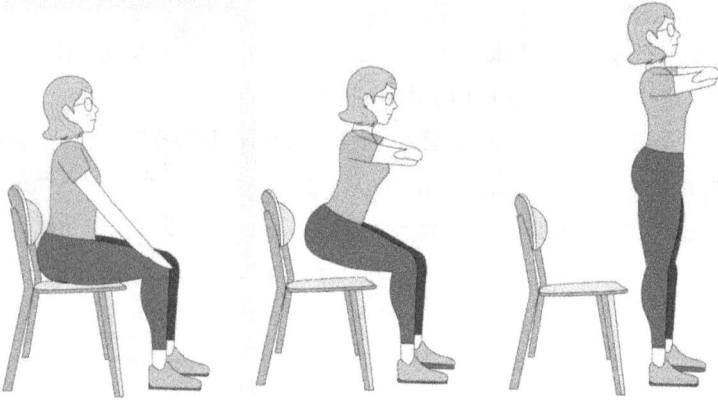

Seated Knee Lift: While sitting upright at the edge of the chair, lift one knee toward your chest while keeping your other foot flat on the ground. Repeating this exercise, alternating legs. This strengthens the thighs and glutes and engages the lower abdominal muscles, supporting core stability. You can loop a lightweight band around your thighs just above the knees for added resistance. The added resistance helps intensify the exercise, further strengthening the muscles.

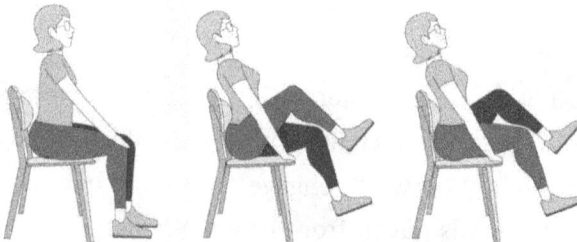

Seated Calf Raises: While sitting upright with back straight and both feet flat on the surface, lift your heels as high as you can while keeping your toes flat. Tighten the muscle and hold for a brief moment, then lower them back down and repeat the process. Over time you can apply some resistance with pressure from your hands on your knees, hold dumbells and something to add a slight bit of weight as you progress.

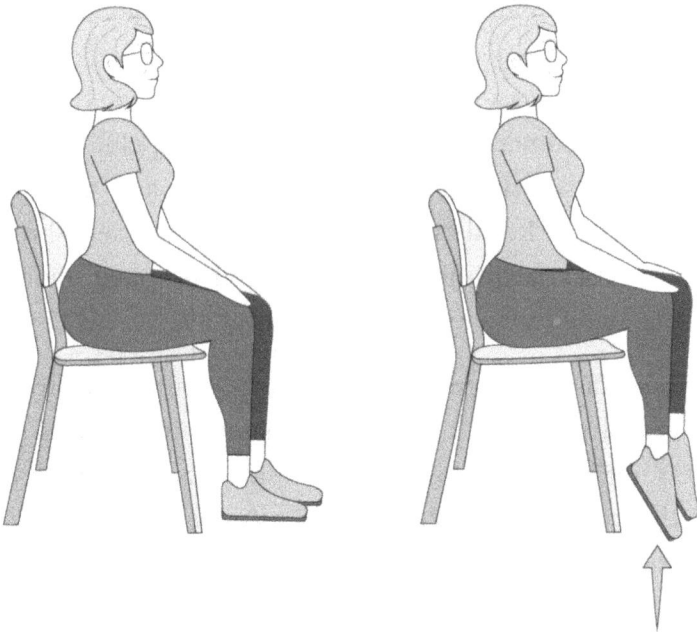

Incorporating exercises that enhance strength and coordination is crucial for overall mobility. The seated side leg raise is an excellent example. While seated, slowly lift one leg out to the side and then bring it back in. This exercise not only strengthens the outer thighs and glutes but also challenges balance and coordination, as maintaining posture while performing the movement requires core engagement.

Introducing variations is vital to keeping your exercise routine engaging and compelling. For example, altering the speed of your leg lifts or adding small ankle weights can vary the intensity and focus of the workout. Performing exercises at a slower pace increases muscle tension and enhances strength, while adding weights provides resistance, boosting muscle growth and endurance.

Strengthening your legs and glutes has substantial real-world benefits. Stronger legs improve your ability to perform daily tasks such as climbing stairs or getting up from a chair. Enhanced muscle strength in these areas also stabilizes your gait, reducing the risk of falls—a common concern for many seniors. Strong glutes support the lower back, alleviating common discomfort and preventing potential injuries. Regularly engaging these muscles through targeted exercises helps maintain independence and mobility, contributing significantly to a higher quality of life.

As we conclude this segment on building lower body strength through seated exercises, it's clear that maintaining leg and glute strength is not just about physical health; it's about enriching your life with the confidence and capability to enjoy day-to-day activities. These exercises lay a foundation for a more active, independent lifestyle, ensuring you continue to move and function at your best.

In the next chapter, we will explore how to integrate flexibility and balance into your routine, further enhancing your ability to move freely and safely. Thus, we will continue our commitment to building a comprehensive exercise regimen that supports your health and well-being. This natural progression from strengthening to improving flexibility ensures that your fitness journey is balanced, holistic, and tailored to your needs as you age.

CHAPTER FIVE

IMPROVING FLEXIBILITY AND BALANCE

I magine waking up each morning with the flexibility to bend and reach through your daily routine without a hint of stiffness or discomfort. For many seniors, enhancing flexibility isn't just about achieving better movement and reclaiming freedom daily. This chapter guides you through gentle stretching exercises that promise to improve your flexibility and significantly bolster your joint health.

5.1 GENTLE STRETCHING: A GUIDE TO INCREASED FLEXIBILITY

Stretching Fundamentals

The act of stretching does more than elongate your muscles—it's vital to maintain your body's agility and ensure your joints remain in full range of motion. As we age, our muscles naturally lose some of their elasticity, and our joints can become less fluid, making once effortless movements feel challenging. A routine of gentle stretches can significantly counteract these effects by enhancing muscle flexibility and lubricating the joints.

One of the primary benefits of maintaining an active stretching routine is the potential reduction in the risk of injuries. Flexible muscles are less prone to strains because they can withstand more physical stress. For you, this means enjoying everyday activities with a lower risk of injuring yourself. Moreover, stretching enhances blood flow to your muscles, giving them a healthy supply of oxygen and nutrients while flushing out waste products. Together, these contribute to better muscle health and faster recovery from muscle fatigue.

Routine Creation

Developing a personalized stretching routine is your next step towards a more supple body. Begin by focusing on major muscle groups that are crucial for your daily activities, including your shoulders, back, hips, thighs, and calves. There are a variety of stretches for each muscle group. Still, the key is to start with what feels comfortable for you and slowly expand your routine to include a broader range of stretches.

For instance, a simple yet effective stretch for your shoulders can be done right from your chair. Extend your arms to the sides with palms facing down, and gently push your arms back until you feel a stretch in your shoulders and chest. Hold this position for about 15-30 seconds before releasing. When performed regularly, such stretches can significantly enhance your upper body flexibility, making tasks like reaching a high shelf or pulling a sweater over your head much more effortless.

Consistency and Patience

The improvements in flexibility won't occur overnight, and it's imperative to approach your stretching routine with patience and consistency. Set a realistic goal that fits into your daily schedule—

stretching for just 10 minutes a day can yield noticeable benefits. The key is to make stretching a regular part of your routine, like having morning coffee or reading the newspaper. Over time, you will see enhancements in your flexibility, translating into smoother and more fluid movements in your everyday life.

Safety Tips

While stretching is generally safe, proper technique is crucial to avoid potential injuries. Here are some tips to ensure you stretch safely:

1. Warm up your muscles slightly before you begin stretching. This can be as simple as walking around your home for a few minutes or gently marching in place.
2. Avoid bouncing or jerky movements. Stretch smoothly, and hold each stretch statically—without movement—for the best results.
3. Never stretch to the point of pain. You should feel a gentle pull in your muscles, but you've pushed too far if it hurts. Back off to a point where you don't feel pain.
4. Breathe freely as you stretch. Avoid holding your breath, which can cause muscle tension, counteracting the stretching benefits.

Interactive Element: Stretching Log

Consider keeping a stretching log to help you keep track of your progress and maintain consistency. This can be a notebook where you record each stretch, how long you held it, and how it felt. Over time, this log will not only serve as a motivational tool, showing you how far you've come, but it can also help you understand your body's rhythms and needs, allowing you to tailor your routine for the best results.

5.2 BALANCE IN A CHAIR: EXERCISES TO FIND YOUR CENTER

Achieving a sense of balance is not solely about maintaining physical stability; it's about harmonizing your body and mind to function optimally. Understanding the mechanics behind balance is critical to mastering exercises that enhance your strength. Every time you stand, sit, or move, your body engages a complex system that includes your muscles, bones, joints, inner ear, and eyes, all coordinated by your brain. This system works continuously to keep you upright and oriented in your environment. When this coordination falters due to age or other factors, exercises specifically designed to challenge and improve your balance are incredibly beneficial.

Chair exercises tailored for balance focus on strengthening the muscles that help stabilize you, such as your core and leg muscles, while enhancing the neural communication pathways used for balance control. A simple but effective exercise is the seated leg lift. While sitting, extend one leg out in front, hold it for a few seconds, and slowly lower it without letting it immediately touch the ground. This exercise forces your core to engage and maintain balance, strengthening crucial muscles. Another excellent exercise is the chair stand, where you sit at the edge of the chair and use your legs and core to stand up, then slowly sit back down. Repeating this motion builds strength in your lower body and core, crucial areas for good balance.

Incorporating exercises that also require mental focus can further enhance your ability to maintain balance. This is where mindfulness techniques come into play. When you perform balance exercises, focus intensely on each movement, paying attention to how your body feels and how different muscles work together to maintain stability. This mindfulness practice improves your concentration and deepens the connection between your mind and body, making your movements more controlled and stable. For instance, while performing a seated toe tap, where you extend your leg and tap your toe on the ground while keeping the rest of your body still, concentrate on the movement of your leg and the slight adjustments your body makes to keep your balance. This focused awareness helps train your brain better to manage your body's balance in the future.

Applying the improved balance to your daily activities transforms these exercises from simple routines to essential life skills. With better balance, the risk of falls decreases significantly, enhancing your safety and independence. Walking up a flight of stairs, stepping off a curb, or navigating through crowded areas becomes more manageable. Moreover, improved balance gives you the confidence to participate more actively in various activities, whether gardening, playing with grandchildren, or enjoying a leisurely walk in the park. This newfound confidence can open up a world of activities that perhaps seemed challenging, enriching your life with more engagement and enjoyment.

As you continue to practice these balance exercises, remember that each session builds your physical stability and confidence in moving through life safely and independently. These exercises are not just about avoiding falls; they're about empowering you to live your life to the fullest, with the assurance that you can handle whatever physical challenges come your way.

5.3 DYNAMIC MOVEMENTS FOR EVERYDAY STABILITY

Incorporating dynamic movements into your chair exercise routine is not just about enhancing your physical capacity; it's about translating these improvements into real-life applications that improve your daily life. Dynamic chair exercises mimic the activities you might perform throughout the day, such as reaching, bending, or twisting. These movements require a certain level of stability and strength, which these exercises aim to build progressively.

Dynamic exercises are particularly beneficial as they prepare you for the various physical challenges, from lifting a grocery bag to more complex movements like bending down to tie your shoes or reaching up to grab something from a high shelf. For example, a dynamic chair exercise might involve simulated rowing motions that engage both your arms and your core and back muscles, mirroring the actions you might use when pulling open a heavy door or drawer. Another exercise could be the seated box pass, where you pass an imaginary box from one side of your body to the other, twisting your torso. This strengthens your core muscles and enhances your ability to perform twisting motions safely and effectively.

Ensuring that the exercises are tailored to your current physical abilities is essential to get the most benefits. If you are starting out or have significant mobility restrictions, you might begin with gentle, minimal-range movements. As your strength and confidence improve, you can gradually increase the intensity and range of motion. This adaptation ensures that the exercises remain challenging yet achievable, providing you with a continual sense of progression and achievement. For instance, if initially lifting your arm to shoulder height is what your mobility allows, start there. Over time, as your flexibility and muscle strength improve, extend your arm above your head to simulate reaching for higher items.

Furthermore, it's crucial to assess how well these exercises are serving your needs frequently. Self-assessment is a valuable tool in this process. After performing these dynamic movements, take a moment to reflect on how you feel. Are there movements that feel too easy or challenging? Are you experiencing discomfort or pain with specific exercises? This feedback is essential for adjusting the exercises to fit your needs better and preventing potential injuries. If a particular movement consistently causes discomfort, modifying it or consulting with a health professional might be necessary to ensure you're performing it correctly and safely.

Dynamic chair exercises are an excellent way to ensure that your exercise routine's benefits extend beyond improved physical health. They significantly impact your ability to perform daily tasks with greater ease and confidence. They enhance your physical stability and build a bridge between your workout and your daily activities, making each movement a step towards a more active and independent lifestyle.

As we close this chapter on improving flexibility and balance, it's clear that the exercises discussed are more than just routines; they are stepping stones to a more vibrant and capable life. Each stretch, balanced hold, and dynamic movement is a building block towards surviving in your environment and thriving within it. This foundation of strength and stability supports your physical health. It enriches your everyday experiences, allowing you to engage with life fully. As we turn the page to the next chapter, we will explore how these foundational elements help us delve deeper into enhancing cardiovascular health, further broadening the scope of your wellness journey.

CHAPTER SIX

CHAIR YOGA FOR MIND AND BODY

I magine your body as a serene temple where peace and energy flow harmoniously. Maintaining this harmony becomes increasingly crucial for our overall well-being as we age. Chair yoga is a gentle but effective way to nurture this balance, combining physical postures with the profound power of breath to rejuvenate the mind and body. This chapter introduces you to the foundational breathing techniques of chair yoga, which are pivotal for enhancing the effectiveness of each pose and fostering a more profound sense of inner calm and vitality in your everyday life.

6.1 BREATHING TECHNIQUES: THE FOUNDATION OF CHAIR YOGA

Breath Awareness

The journey into chair yoga begins with understanding and mastering your breath. Breath, or 'Prana' as it is known in yogic philosophy, is the vital life force that energizes every cell of our body. Learning to control and deepen this vital force through breathing techniques can transform your health, offering every-thing from enhanced relaxation to improved energy levels.

Breathing exercises, or 'Pranayama,' teach us to breathe through the diaphragm, allowing for full oxygen exchange that can boost the efficiency of your lungs and profoundly relax the mind. The prac-tice typically starts with observing your natural breath. This might seem simple, but it's a powerful exercise to ground your awareness and connect deeply with your current state. Try this: sit comfortably in your chair with your back straight and hands on your knees. Please close your eyes and take a moment to notice your breath without trying to change it. Feel the air flowing through your nostrils, the gentle rise and lowering of your chest or stomach. This mindful observation is the first step in developing breath aware-ness. This skill enhances your ability to focus and calms your mind.

Pranayama Practices

Once familiar with observing your breath, you can explore specific Pranayama practices. One such practice adapted for chair yoga is the 'Dirga Pranayama,' or three-part breath. This technique involves deeply inhaling into your abdomen and ribcage and then into your chest and reversing the order during exhalation. This complete and conscious way of breathing can dramatically increase your lung capacity, improve respiratory functions, and instill a sense of calm throughout your nervous system.

Another adapted practice is 'Nadi Shodhana,' or alternate nostril breathing. This involves holding one nostril closed while breathing through the other and switching sides. This practice effectively balances the body's energies and calms the mind. It also helps reduce stress and enhance mental clarity.

Integration with Movement

Integrating these breathing techniques into chair yoga poses increases their physical and mental health benefits. For example, when performing a seated spinal twist, coordinating your breath with your movements—inhaling as you lengthen your spine and exhaling as you deepen into the twist—can enhance the stretch and relaxation effects. This combination helps maintain an even flow of energy. It keeps you deeply connected to the present moment, enhancing your mindfulness and the overall yoga experience.

Daily Breathing Routines

Including these breathing exercises in your daily routine will be an effective tool for managing stress and boosting your mood. Taking just a few minutes daily to practice Pranayama can help regulate your body's stress response, improve your sleep quality, and elevate your overall well-being. Consider beginning your day with five minutes of 'Dirga Pranayama' to invigorate your body and mind or winding down in the evening with a few rounds of 'Nadi Shodhana' to promote a restful night's sleep.

Interactive Element: Breathing Log

Consider maintaining a breathing log to help you cultivate a regular Pranayama practice. Each day, jot down which techniques you practiced, how long you spent on each, and any feelings or sensations you experienced during and after the practice. This log will not only serve as a motivational tool, reminding you of the profound benefits these practices offer, but it will also provide insightful reflections on how Pranayama affects your body and mind over time.

Breath is not just fundamental to life; it is a cornerstone of wellness in yoga. By mastering the art of breathing, you not only enhance your chair yoga practice but also equip yourself with a powerful tool to navigate the complexities of aging with grace and vitality. As you continue to explore these techniques, remember that every breath brings you closer to a more balanced, energized, and harmonious state of being.

6.2 RELAXATION AND MEDITATION: MINDFUL MOVEMENTS IN A CHAIR

The gentle sway of a calm sea, the whisper of the wind in the trees —nature effortlessly teaches us the art of relaxation and meditation. In chair yoga, these principles are brought into your daily practice, transforming simple movements and stillness into a profound experience of peace and well-being. As we explore the serene world of meditation and relaxation from the comfort of our chairs, we find tools for managing stress and enriching our lives with a more profound sense of calm and presence.

While seated in a chair, meditation opens up a world of mindfulness that can be especially beneficial as we navigate the later years of life. A simple practice involves focusing on a single, calming image or thought. Picture a scene from nature, a quiet lake at dawn, or a starry sky. As you hold this image in your mind, let your body begin to relax, your breathing deepens, and your thoughts pass like leaves on a breezy day. This technique, known as guided imagery meditation, will not only help reduce stress but also enhance the ability to concentrate and stay present in the moment. Another effective meditation technique for chair yoga is the body scan. Starting from the tips of your toes and moving slowly up to the crown of your head, mentally scan your body for areas of discomfort or tension. As you pinpoint these areas, picture your breath flowing into them, releasing the tension with each exhale. This practice promotes relaxation and fosters a heightened awareness of your body's sensations, which can be particularly beneficial for identifying and addressing discomfort before it escalates.

The connection between your mind and body is a powerful conduit for health and well-being, and chair yoga offers unique opportunities to strengthen this connection. Each pose and movement in chair yoga invites physical and mental engagement. For instance, when practicing a seated twist, focus not only on the movement of your spine but also on the sensation of release and opening that the twist brings. Engage your mind by being fully present in the moment, feeling each muscle as it stretches, and observing any emotional responses you might have. This mindful engagement helps deepen the exercise's impact, turning a simple physical stretch into a holistic practice that nurtures mental and emotional health.

Relaxation techniques designed explicitly for chair yoga can further enhance your practice and provide immediate relief from stress. Progressive muscle relaxation involves tensing and then relaxing different muscle groups. This can be particularly effective while seated, allowing you to focus intensely on each area. Begin by tensing the muscles in your feet, hold for a few seconds, and then release. Methodically work your way up through your legs, torso, arms, and head. As you release the tension from your muscles, imagine it melting away, leaving your body relaxed and calm. Another simple but powerful relaxation exercise is the palm press. Bring your palms together in front of your chest and press them firmly against each other for a few seconds, then release. Repeat this several times, using the pressure to help release any built-up tension. These practices help reduce physical stress and calm the mind, making them perfect for integrating into your regular chair yoga routine.

To make the most of these relaxation and meditation practices:

1. Consider integrating them into your daily chair yoga routine.
2. Start your session with a few minutes of guided imagery to settle your mind and prepare your body for the physical exercises.
3. Incorporate mindful movement into each yoga pose, focusing intensely on the sensations and emotions that each pose evokes.
4. End your session with a body scan or progressive muscle relaxation to leave your practice feeling profoundly relaxed and rejuvenated.

Over time, these practices will enhance your chair yoga experience and contribute to a greater sense of peace and well-being in your everyday life. As you continue to explore and integrate these techniques, remember that each moment of mindfulness and relaxation is a precious gift to your overall health, one that enriches your physical state and your mental and emotional landscape.

6.3 YOGA POSES ADAPTED FOR CHAIR PRACTICE

One of the most extraordinary aspects of yoga is its adaptability to different needs and circumstances, allowing everyone to benefit from its practices. In chair yoga, traditional poses are modified to make them accessible to individuals who may find it challenging to perform floor-based exercises. These adaptations ensure that everyone can enjoy yoga's physical, mental, and emotional benefits regardless of mobility level. Let's explore how you can adapt common yoga poses for chair practice, create an engaging sequence, and achieve a balance between enhancing flexibility and building strength.

Transforming traditional yoga poses into chair-based exercises allows individuals to practice yoga safely and comfortably. For example, the classic 'Cat-Cow' stretch, typically performed on hands and knees, can be adapted to a seated version. You sit forward in your chair, place your hands on your knees, and alternate between arching your back and rounding it, mimicking the cat and cow movements. This adaptation helps loosen the spine and relieve back tension while safely seated. Another fundamental pose, the 'Warrior,' can also be modified for chair practice. Instead of standing, you sit and extend one leg out to the side, turning your torso towards the extended leg and raising your arms, maintaining the strong, warrior stance. These adaptations maintain the essence and benefits of the original poses and ensure they are inclusive.

Creating a flowing sequence of chair yoga poses enhances the enjoyment and effectiveness of your practice. Begin with gentle warm-up movements, such as shoulder rolls and neck stretches, to prepare your body. Progress to more dynamic stretching poses like the adapted 'Cat-Cow' to further loosen up. Gradually include strength-building poses such as the seated 'Warrior' or 'Chair Pigeon,' where you cross one ankle over the opposite thigh and gently lean forward to stretch the hip. Finally, wind down with slower, deeper stretches and a quiet time of reflection or meditation to conclude your session. This sequence allows for a holistic practice that warms up the body, engages significant muscle groups, and then brings focus and calm, mimicking the natural energy flow of traditional yoga practices.

Balancing the practice to enhance flexibility and muscular strength is crucial for a holistic approach to chair yoga. While flexibility exercises help maintain joint health and ease of movement, strength exercises fortify muscles and bones, enhancing overall stability and stamina. For instance, alternating between a flexibility-focused pose like the seated 'Forward Bend' and a strength-focused pose like the seated 'Twist' can provide a balanced workout. The 'Forward Bend' encourages spinal and hamstring flexibility, while the 'Twist' strengthens the abdominal and back muscles by requiring you to hold your position against the twist. All of these yoga poses will be extremely beneficial.

Cat-Cow: Sit upright with spine straight and your feet flat, shoulder width apart. Place your hands on your knees. When you exhale, round your spine and bring your chin to your chest. Have a few relaxed breaths while in this position. Then exhale while gradually bringing your head up and back to the upright position.

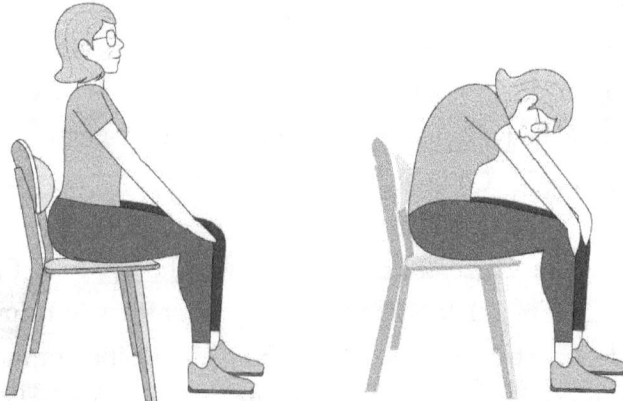

<u>Spinal Twist</u>: Start by turning sideways in your chair, facing your right. While exhaling lift your spine and start twisting your torso to the right, you may hold on to the chair back. While inhaling try to lengthen your spine from your seat to your head, like your lifting your body away from the chair without actually getting up. During your exhaling try to deepen the stretch slightly further. Perform this 4 to 5 times. Then bring your body back to the front and repeat stretch on the left side.

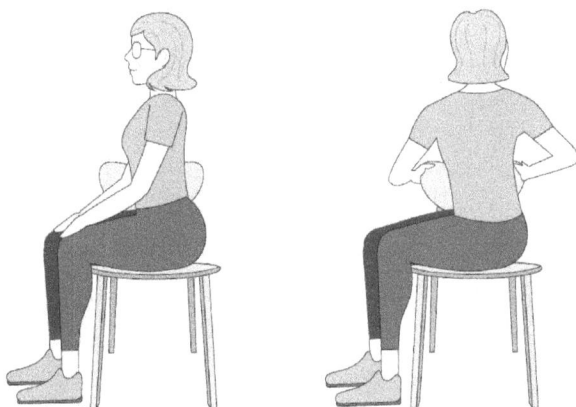

<u>Warrior I</u>: Sit upright with spine straight and your feet flat, shoulder width apart. Now, shift towards the left edge of the chair. The left leg is out towards the left. Form a 90-degree angle with your knee so that it aligns with your ankle and hip. Keep foot flat, with the toes pointed left. Inhale and bring your right foot back as far as possible, extending it straight back on your toes. Inhale, then while you exhale raise your hands so they clasp over your head. Enterlaced with your pointers and thumbs out toward the ceiling. Shoul-

ders relaxed from your ears and allow them to slide down your back. Inhale and exhale deeply several times, then while exhaling unclasp your fingers and allow your arms to gently go back to your sides. Then gently slide your back leg to the front and preposition yourself to perform on the other side.

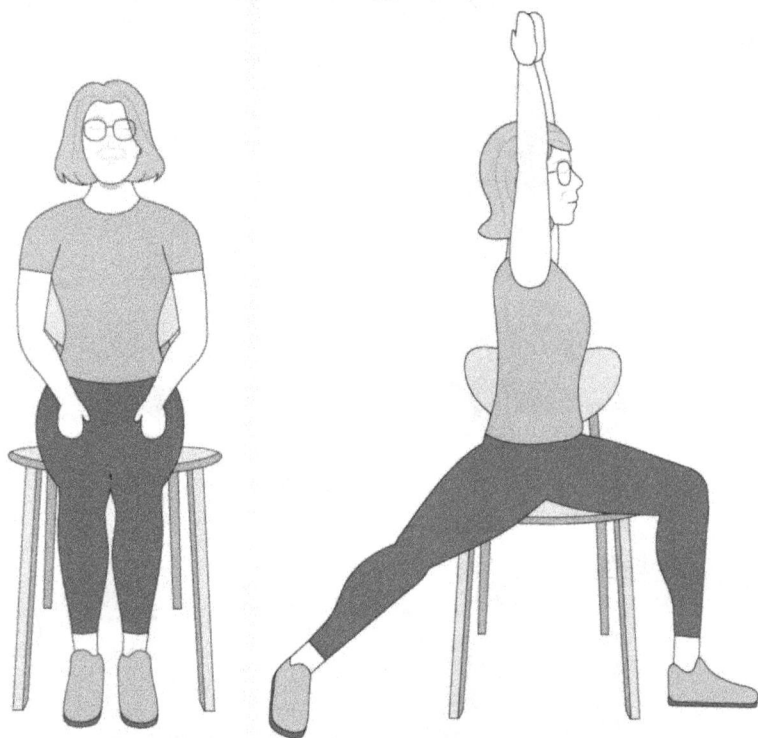

<u>Tree Pose</u>: Sit upright at the edge of the chair. Inhale deeply, expanding your chest and lower your shoulder blades downward. Keep your head straight forward and bring your left leg straight in front of you. Flex your foot with your toes toward the floor. Bring your right leg out to the side, keeping your knee bent and your toes on the floor. Bring your hands together in a prayer position by your

heart or you can stretch them to the ceiling. Take a few breaths and then gradually bring your right leg back and have both feet planted flat in front of you. Then come back to starting position and repeat with the other side.

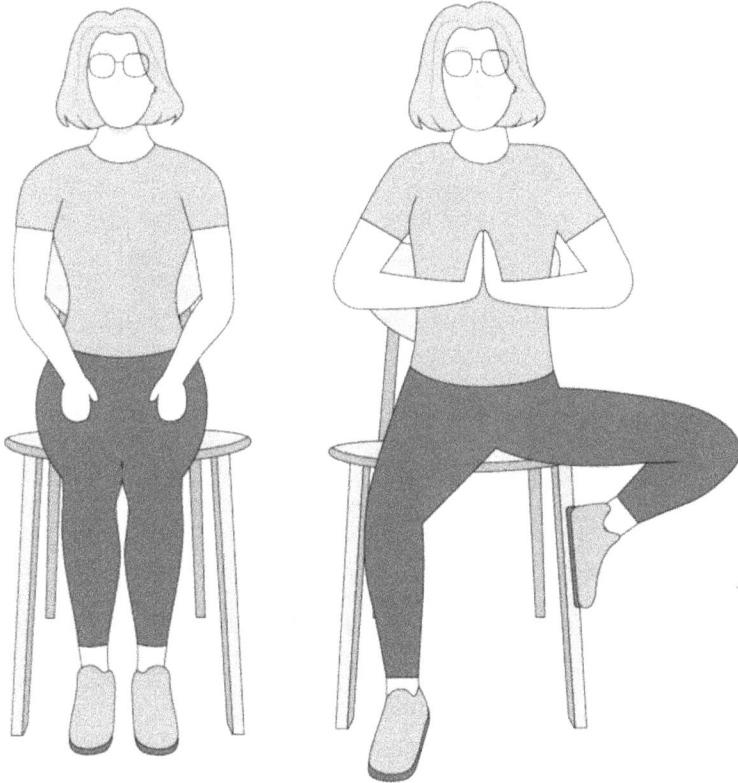

Eagle Arms: While sitting in the upright position inhale and stretch your arms to the side. Then as your exhale bring your arms around the front and overlapping. Continue until you are able to grab your opposite shoulder, like a self hug. Try to reach around as far as comfortably possible. Then inhale and raise your elbows up a couple inches. When you exhale allow your shoulders to drop down and away from your ears. Take several deep breaths while repeating raise and lowering technique.

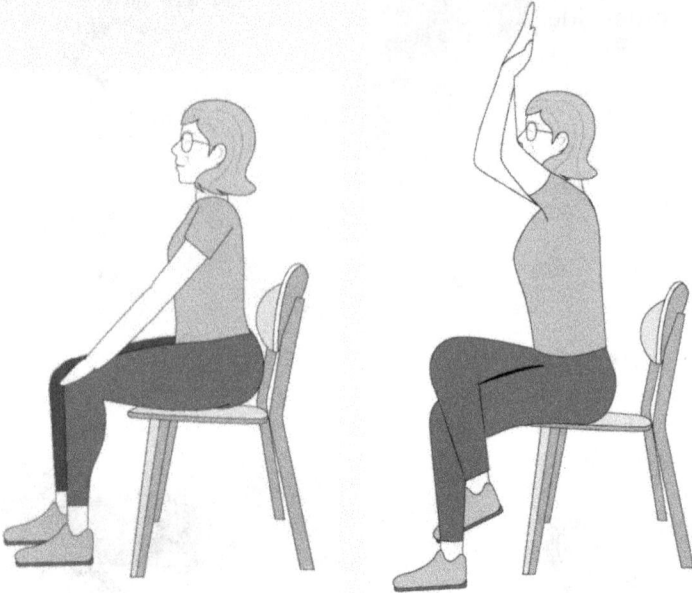

Extended Triangle Pose: Sit with your body to the right side of the chair so that your right thigh clears the seat. Then bring your right leg out to your side while trying to straighten as much as possible. Inhale and bring your arms straight out in front and parallel to the floor. Ensure that your palms face down and keep your shoulders wide. Exhale and while bending from your hip, lean your body toward your right leg. Place your right hand on your right thigh or shin and bring your left arm straight up toward the ceiling. You can either keep your head straight, turn toward your left hand or facing ther floor. Take some deep breaths then inhale and gradually return to the starting position. Repeat on the side.

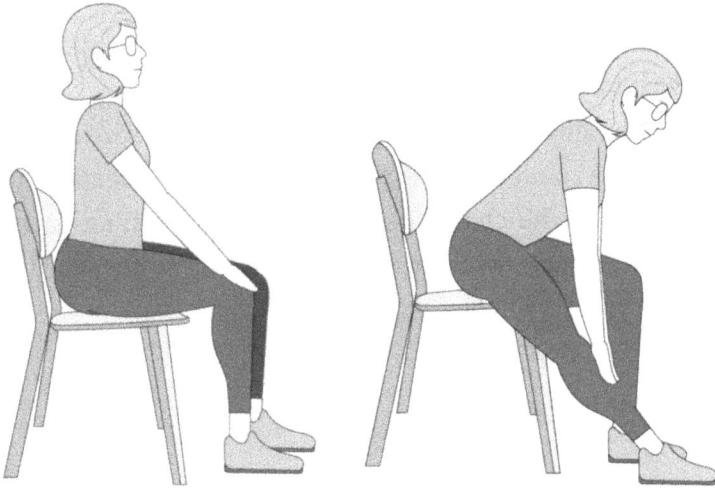

Single Leg Stretch: While sitting upright at the edge of the chair, stretch one leg out with heel on the floor and toes upward. If your leg is not straight then get as close to the seat edge as safely possible. Have both hands resting on the outstretched leg. Inhale upward and as you begin to exhale start to bend over your outstretched leg while reaching down your leg as far as you comfortably can. Do not force the stretch, then grab a hold of the furthest part you can reach and take several relaxed deep breaths. On the last exhale gradually return to the upright position. Repeat with the other leg while still ensuring good balance and support on the chair.

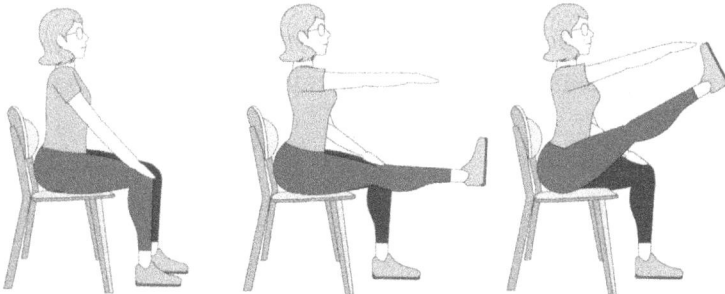

<u>Half Lord of the Fishes</u>: While sitting upright bring your left leg over your right leg. Inhale and bring both arms straight up. Exhale and twist to your left while bringing your hands down to grab the back of the chair. Then gradually turn your head over your left shoulder to a comfortable neck stretch. Take a few deep breaths and then let go of the chair; then inhale while reaching back to the ceiling and exhale while gradually returning to the starting position. Then repeat on the right side.

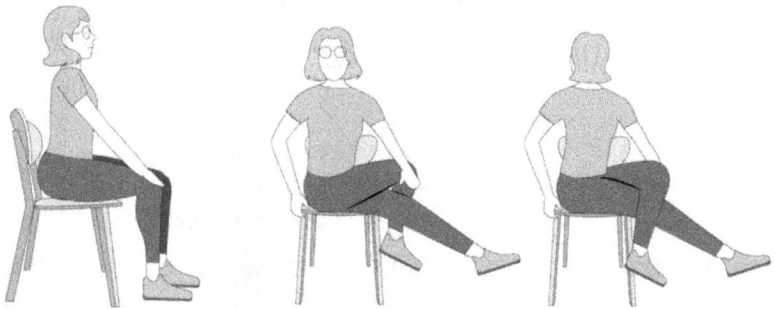

<u>Marichyasana III</u>: Sitting upright being supported by the chair back and with your feet flat, shoulder width apart. Bring your right knee to your chest and place that foot on the front of the chair seat as close to your buttucks as possible. Inhale upward, straightening your spine; Exhale and twist to the right. Reach around your right knee with your left hand and clasp your right hand. Take a few deep breaths. With each deep inhalation straighten upright and slightly twist a touch more with your exhale. Release and gradually go back to the neutral starting position. Repeat with the left leg.

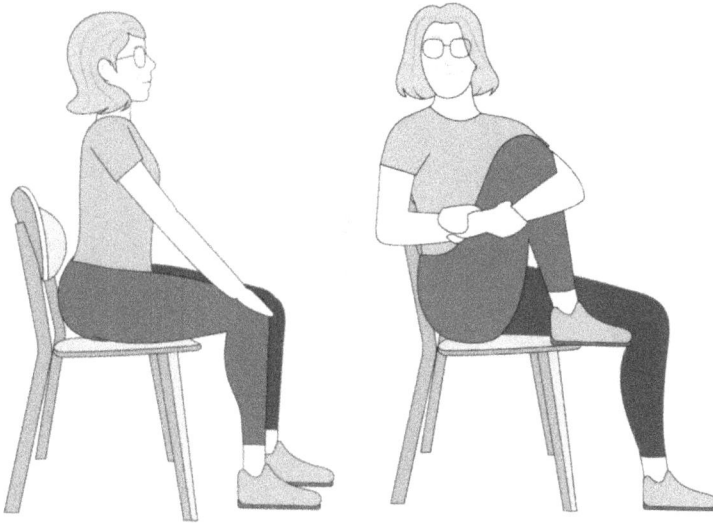

Chair Downward-Facing Dog: Have the chair facing away so that the back is toward you. Position your body directly behind the chair an arms length away with feet shoulder width apart. Then bend from your hips, keep your back straight and place your hands on the outsides of the chair back. Gradually bring your feet back until your arms are fully extended. Slide your hands down the sides while your doing this to allow stability. Keep your heels firmly on the floor and hold this position as long as comfortably possible. Then gradually bring your feet forward and raise your body back upright.

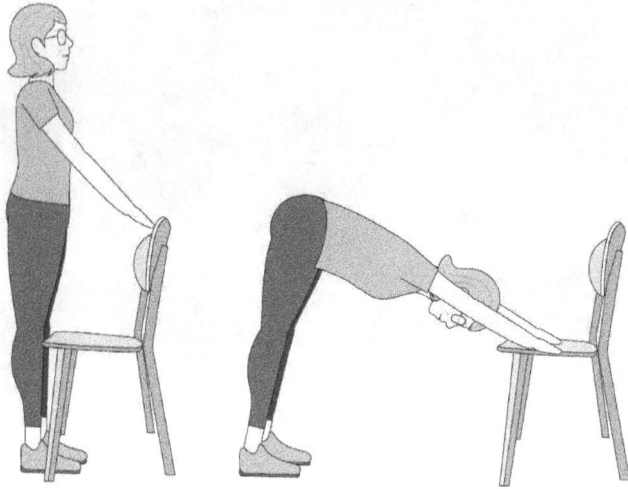

Discussing the holistic benefits of chair yoga reveals its potential to enhance quality of life significantly. Regular practice can improve posture, as many adapted poses focus on alignment and muscle balance. This can reduce common age-related issues such as back pain and stiffness. Anxiety reduction is another profound benefit, as mindful breathing and slow movements help calm the mind, reduce stress, and promote emotional balance. Additionally, chair yoga enhances body awareness, helping you become more attuned to your body's needs and rhythms, leading to better overall health management and a more active lifestyle.

In summary, chair yoga makes the rich benefits of traditional yoga accessible to everyone by adapting poses for chair use, creating sequences that enhance both flexibility and strength and addressing holistic health needs. This practice improves physical health and enriches emotional and mental well-being, making it a great addition to your wellness routine. As we transition from the rejuvenating practices of chair yoga, we will explore enhancing cardiovascular health through chair exercises, continuing our focus on building a comprehensive, health-promoting, enjoyable, and sustainable lifestyle.

CHAPTER SEVEN
BOOSTING CARDIOVASCULAR HEALTH

W hen you think of cardiovascular health, your mind might immediately picture vigorous jogging or cycling. However, maintaining a healthy heart can mean something other than high-impact activities that may be challenging or unsuitable for your current fitness level. Chair exercises provide a fantastic alternative, allowing you to boost your heart health gently and enjoyably right from your seat. This chapter will introduce you to the delightful world of chair marching, a simple yet effective way to get your heart pumping and blood flowing while ensuring your comfort and safety.

7.1 THE JOY OF CHAIR MARCHING: AN INTRODUCTION TO CARDIO

Simple Start: Chair Marching as an Accessible Way to Begin Cardio Workouts

Chair marching is an excellent entry point into cardiovascular exercise, especially if you're embarking on your fitness journey or standing exercises are not feasible. This activity involves marching in place while seated, lifting your knees alternately in a rhythmic fashion. It's a movement that mimics walking or marching but with the added stability and support of sitting. You can adjust the intensity according to your comfort and capability, making it an inclusive exercise suitable for varying fitness levels.

The beauty of chair marching lies in its simplicity and adaptability. You can start with just a few minutes per session and gradually increase as your endurance improves. This exercise helps elevate your heart rate, promoting better blood circulation and health. Moreover, it engages multiple muscle groups, providing a comprehensive workout that benefits your cardiovascular system and strengthens your legs and core.

Heart Rate Monitoring: Techniques to Monitor Heart Rate During Exercise

Monitoring your heart rate during exercise is crucial to ensure you work within a safe and effective range. It helps you gauge the intensity of your workout and make necessary adjustments to optimize benefits while avoiding strain. Maintaining an appropriate heart rate is particularly important for seniors to prevent overexertion.

You can monitor your heart rate manually by placing two fingers (not your thumb) on your wrist or the side of your neck to feel your pulse. Count the number of beats in 15 seconds and multiply by four to get your beats per minute. Alternatively, a digital heart rate monitor or a smartwatch can provide a more convenient and accurate reading. These devices can also alert you if your heart rate exceeds recommended limits, ensuring you maintain a safe intensity level.

Incremental Increases: How to Gradually Increase Intensity and Duration to Improve Cardiovascular Health Without Strain

To get the most from your chair marching and other cardiovascular activities, gradually increase the intensity and duration of your workouts. Incremental increases help your body adapt safely without undue stress, reducing the risk of injury or cardiovascular complications.

Start with what feels manageable—perhaps marching slowly for five minutes. As this becomes easier, you can increase the duration in small increments, such as an additional minute every few sessions. To enhance intensity, try lifting your knees higher, increasing the speed of your march, or incorporating arm movements, like reaching up or swinging your arms. These minor adjustments keep the exercise challenging and ensure continued improvement in your cardiovascular health.

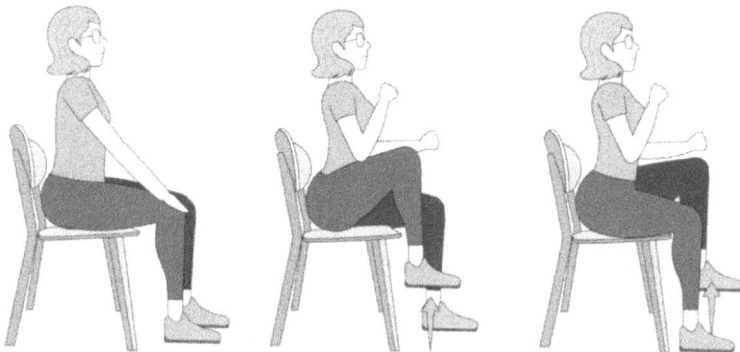

Chair Marching: Sitting upright, slowly lift one knee towards your chest while keeping your abdominal muscles tight, then lower it and repeat with the other knee. This exercise warms up your core muscles and gently engages your lower back and hips. Start with 30 seconds and continue to increase as your cardio improves.

<u>Seated Arm Circles</u>: While sitting upright, extend your arms straight out to the sides. Begin to rotate your arms forward in small circles for 30 seconds, then you will switch and rotate backward in small circles for 30 seconds. Once you have mastered this exercise you can repeat it and make larger circles on the 2nd set.

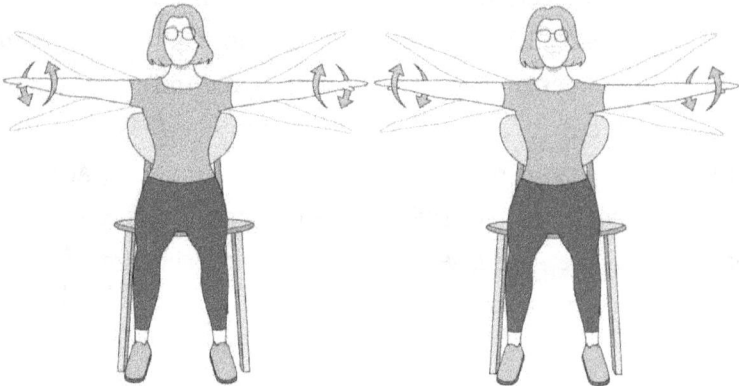

<u>Seated Burpee</u>: Sit upright with spine straight and your feet flat, shoulder width apart, arms at your sides. Begin by engaging your core, lift your arms straight up over your head and allow your shoulders go back and down. Swiftly lower your arms to your thighs, then bend forward at your hips trying to touch your chest to your thighs while reaching your arms toward the floor in front of your feet. If your are able you can tap the floor. Then immediately perform the steps in reverse. Do 10 reps for 1 set to start.

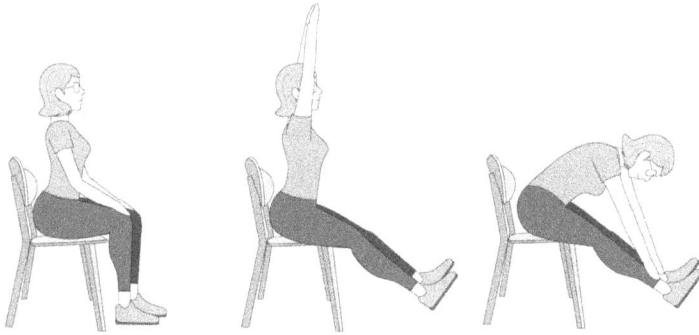

Engagement and Enjoyment: Keeping the Routine Enjoyable with Music and Variation to Encourage Regular Practice

Maintaining motivation is crucial in sustaining any exercise regimen. Making your workout enjoyable is one of the most effective ways to ensure you look forward to and consistently engage in your exercise sessions. Integrating music into your chair marching routine can significantly enhance the enjoyment factor. Choose tunes that uplift your spirits and match the rhythm you wish to maintain during exercise. Music makes the activity more enjoyable but can also help you maintain a steady pace, making your workout more effective.

Additionally, introducing variations can keep the routine fresh and exciting. Alternate the pace, change the height of your knee lifts, or add different arm movements to create a dance-like sequence. These variations not only prevent boredom but also challenge different muscle groups, enhancing the overall effectiveness of your workout.

Interactive Element: Reflective Journaling Prompt

Consider keeping a reflective journal to further engage with your exercise routine and track your progress. After each session, jot down how you felt during the exercise, any changes in your endurance or strength, and your emotional response to the workout. Reflecting on these entries can provide insights into how your body responds to the exercises and help you tailor your routine to meet your fitness and health goals. This practice encourages a mindful approach to exercise, where you're improving your physical health and becoming more attuned to your body's needs and responses.

Incorporating chair marching into your routine is a beautiful way to enhance your cardiovascular health in a manner that respects your body's limits while providing ample opportunity for enjoyment and personal growth. As you continue to explore and expand your cardiovascular exercises, remember that each step, no matter how small, is a positive stride towards a healthier heart and a more vibrant life.

7.2 SEATED DANCE MOVES: COMBINING FUN AND FITNESS

In the dynamic spectrum of chair exercises to enhance cardiovascular health, seated dance emerges as a delightful and effective method of merging rhythm and movement. This form of exercise transcends traditional fitness routines by infusing dance movements into the seated exercise regime, making it a physical activity and an expression of cultural heritage and personal creativity. Seated dance leverages dance's natural joy and rhythmic engagement to maintain heart health, making it an appealing option for those who might find other forms of exercise monotonous or physically daunting.

Rhythmic exercise such as seated dance is particularly beneficial because it combines music and coordinated movements to elevate heart rate in a joyful, stimulating manner. Following a rhythm helps to synchronize your movements, enhancing cardiovascular health and rhythmic coordination and timing, which are essential cognitive skills. As you move to the beat, each dance sequence encourages your heart to pump faster, circulating blood more effectively throughout your body and improving overall heart function. The inherent flexibility of dance allows you to adjust the intensity as per your comfort, ensuring that you receive the optimal cardiovascular benefits without strain.

The variety of dance movements inspired by different cultures adds an enriching layer to this exercise format. Each culture offers unique dance styles incorporating different movements, rhythms, and postures, providing a rich tapestry of options to explore. For instance, a seated version of the flamenco can introduce you to the vigorous hand clapping and intricate wrist twirls of Spanish dance. In contrast, an adapted Bollywood dance routine can immerse you in the dramatic expressions and vibrant motions typical of Indian cinema. Engaging with these diverse dance forms keeps the exercise routine engaging and colorful. It fosters a deeper appreciation and connection to various cultural heritages. This diversity can transform your exercise routine into a global exploration, where each session brings a new cultural experience, keeping the routine fresh and exciting.

Participating in group dance sessions, whether in person or virtually, adds a valuable social dimension to your exercise routine. Even through a screen, dancing together can create a sense of community and shared joy, often lacking in solitary workout regimes. These group interactions can be particularly uplifting, providing motivation to engage regularly and offering emotional support and camaraderie. For many, connecting with others over fun activities like dancing can significantly enhance the enjoyment and anticipation of exercise sessions. It transforms the routine from a solitary health task into a social event to look forward to, filled with laughter, music, and mutual encouragement.

Beyond the cardiovascular benefits and social enjoyment, seated dance also significantly enhances cognitive functions such as memory and coordination. Learning and remembering dance sequences stimulates the brain, improving memory capacity and mental agility. The coordination required to synchronize your movements with the music and sequence further challenges your brain, fostering neural connectivity and motor skills. This cognitive engagement is a crucial aspect of aging healthily, as it helps keep your mind sharp and alert, complementing the physical benefits of exercise with mental and neurological health advantages.

As you continue to explore the vibrant world of seated dance, each session enriches your fitness journey with rhythm, cultural exploration, social interaction, and cognitive engagement. This holistic approach enhances your physical health and nurtures your mental and emotional well-being, making seated dance a profoundly enriching component of your cardiovascular health regimen. As you sway, tap, and move to the rhythms of diverse cultures, remember that each step is not just a move towards better physical health but also a step towards a more joyful, connected, and vibrant life.

7.3 CARDIO CIRCUIT: ROTATING THROUGH HEART-HEALTHY EXERCISES

Creating a cardio circuit that rotates through various heart-healthy exercises offers an engaging and effective way to enhance cardiovascular health. This method involves designing a series of exercises you perform sequentially, each targeting different aspects of cardiovascular fitness. The beauty of a cardio circuit lies in its structured yet dynamic nature, allowing for an optimized workout that maintains your interest and pushes your fitness levels without overwhelming you.

The setup of your cardio circuit should include a variety of exercises that can be performed while seated or with the chair as support. For example, you might start with arm circles for upper body warming, followed by seated leg lifts, then move on to more intense chair marches and conclude with gentle stretches. Arranging these exercises in a sequence ensures that you engage different muscle groups and maintain a steady heart rate elevation throughout the session. The key is to balance intensity and recovery. While one exercise might raise your heart rate, the next could allow for slight recovery, preparing you for the next bout of intensity. This alternation helps maximize cardiovascular benefits while reducing the risk of fatigue.

Managing time within your circuit is crucial, especially when beginning your fitness journey. Each exercise in your circuit should be timed to ensure you maintain focus and intensity without risking overexertion. Beginners might start with one minute per exercise interval, with equal rest periods in between. As your endurance improves, you can gradually increase the exercise time and reduce the rest intervals. Keeping each session timed helps you stay on track and ensures that your workout remains manageable. A simple timer or a stopwatch can be an invaluable tool during these workouts, helping you keep precise track of your exercise and rest periods.

Progress tracking is another essential element of maintaining a successful cardio-circuit routine. Monitoring your improvements in cardiovascular health can be incredibly motivating and informative. You might track how many repetitions of a particular exercise you can perform in a set time as your stamina increases or note how quickly your heart rate returns to normal after a session, an indicator of your cardiovascular recovery rate. These metrics can be recorded in a workout journal or tracked using a fitness app, providing concrete data on your progress. Over time, this data shows your improvements and helps you adjust your routine to keep challenging your cardiovascular system effectively.

Adaptability in your cardio circuit ensures that the exercises remain appropriate for your health needs and fitness level. This might mean modifying specific movements to reduce strain or adjusting the intensity to match your current capabilities. For instance, if rapid arm movements raise your heart rate too quickly, you could switch to slower, more controlled motions that maintain your heart rate within a safer range. Similarly, if exercise becomes too easy, you might add light weights or increase your speed to continue challenging yourself. Listening to your body and adjusting your routine is vital to maintaining a safe and beneficial workout program.

The circuit approach to cardiovascular exercise keeps your workouts varied and exciting. It ensures comprehensive health benefits that contribute to your overall fitness and well-being. As you continue engaging with these dynamic routines, remember that each rotation boosts your heart health and enhances your endurance, strength, and flexibility, paving the way for a more active and independent lifestyle.

The following are a few YouTube Videos that offer very good workout routines if you get bored with the same cardio exercises. Just get online and plug in the URL or if possible click on the link. You can choose one day a week that you try something new or different. If your going to start a different video you find, you should review the whole thing prior to your workout so that you are prepared.

Beginners Seated HIIT workout for Seniors: https://youtu.be/s5FNlnEuux4?si=uzqHlYraWflUwfNx

10 minute chair exercise:

https://youtu.be/9PpO-sh2HD4?si=cw-J54pZ1SyfLfVi

10 minutes chair exercises for beginners:

https://youtu.be/mevvQo3uHFU?si=2BLgFHcO3rgbqL–

As we conclude this chapter on enhancing cardiovascular health through chair exercises, it's clear that the journey towards a healthier heart can be both enjoyable and deeply rewarding. From the rhythmic fun of chair dancing to the structured challenge of cardio circuits, each method offers unique benefits and keeps your routine fresh and engaging. These exercises are more than just movements; they are stepping stones to a heart-healthy lifestyle that promotes longevity and enhances your quality of life. As you move forward, remember that each step, no matter how small, is a victory in your health journey. Next, we will explore how chair exercises can be tailored for those with specific health conditions, ensuring everyone can engage in safe and effective physical activity.

CHAPTER EIGHT

TAILORING EXERCISES FOR HEALTH CONDITIONS

Navigating through life with a health condition can sometimes feel like moving against the current in a river that should be effortlessly carrying you forward. Particularly for those living with arthritis, finding ways to maintain mobility and manage pain can be crucial to the quality of daily life. This chapter delves into how chair exercises can be specifically adapted to accommodate and benefit individuals with arthritis, enhancing joint flexibility and managing pain without exacerbating the condition.

8.1 CHAIR EXERCISES FOR THOSE WITH ARTHRITIS

Gentle Mobility: Introducing Movements that Enhance Joint Flexibility Without Causing Pain

Arthritis often brings with it a reduction in joint flexibility, leading to stiffness and discomfort that can hinder everyday activities. Incorporating gentle mobility exercises into your routine can significantly alleviate these symptoms. Chair exercises designed for arthritis focus on smooth, flowing movements that enhance the range of motion without overstraining the joints. For example, simple chair exercises such as <u>Ankle Circles</u> improve lower body circulation and mobility. Sitting comfortably, extend one leg and rotate the ankle slowly; this not only aids in keeping the joint limber but also stimulates fluid movement within the joint capsule, essential for nourishing the joint and reducing stiffness.

Similarly, <u>Wrist & Finger Stretches</u> can be immensely beneficial, primarily if your arthritis affects your hands. Extend your arm forward in a relaxed manner and gently pull back on each finger and then the entire hand, promoting flexibility in the small joints of the fingers and wrists. You can perform these exercises several times throughout the day. It will help keep joints flexible and functional, encouraging the synovial fluid to keep them well-lubricated and pain at bay.

Pain Management: Techniques and Exercises that Help Manage Arthritis Pain Through Controlled Movements

The cornerstone of managing arthritis pain through exercise is the consistency of low-impact activities that keep the joints moving without causing discomfort. Controlled movements, such as <u>Seated Leg Extensions</u>, can strengthen the muscles around the knees to provide better support for the joints and reduce the load they carry during daily activities. To perform this exercise, sit with your back straight and extend one leg in front of you as far as possible, then slowly lower it back down. This exercise strengthens the quadriceps, which are crucial for knee health.

Implementing controlled breathing techniques alongside these exercises will also play a prominent role in pain management. Deep, mindful breathing can help reduce pain perception and foster a relaxation response, which may decrease inflammation and discomfort.

Joint Protection: Strategies for Exercising that Protect Vulnerable Joints, Including How to Modify Movements to Reduce Strain

Protecting the joints during exercise is paramount for individuals with arthritis. One effective strategy is to use adaptive equipment to modify exercises. For instance, using a chair with excellent back support can help maintain proper posture during exercises, reducing undue stress on the spine and hip joints. Furthermore, incorporating soft grips or wraps around the handles of resistance bands can make them easier to hold if hand arthritis is a concern, thus protecting the finger joints from strain.

Always ensure that your movements are within a comfortable range for your joints. Avoid any motion that causes sharp pain or feels forced. The goal is to enhance mobility and strength without pushing the joints beyond their safe limits.

Warm-Up and Cool-Down: The Critical Role of Proper Warm-Up and Cool-Down Sessions to Prepare the Body for Exercise and Prevent Stiffness Post-Exercise

Proper warm-up and cool-down periods are crucial for beginning and ending your exercise session, especially when dealing with arthritis. A good warm-up prepares the joints by slowly increasing circulation to the muscles and joints, making them more pliable and less prone to injury. Simple seated marches or arm raises can increase your heart rate and adequately warm your body.

Cool-downs are just as important because they help gradually reduce the heart rate and stretch out the muscles you've used during your exercise, preventing stiffness. Gentle stretching or even sitting quietly and practicing deep breathing can be an effective cool-down, helping to consolidate the gains from your workout and minimize any post-exercise soreness or stiffness.

Integrating these tailored chair exercises into your daily routine will help manage arthritis symptoms more effectively. It can also improve your overall mobility and quality of life. They are created to meet you where you are, providing pain relief and improved joint function without risking further discomfort or injury.

8.2 SAFE MOVEMENTS FOR SENIORS WITH OSTEOPOROSIS

Osteoporosis presents unique challenges, particularly when maintaining an active lifestyle without risking bone health. The condition, characterized by decreased bone density and increased fragility, necessitates a careful approach to exercise. Engaging in activities that support bone strengthening without imposing undue stress is crucial. Resistance training and weight-bearing movements, when adapted for chair exercises, provide a safe method to support bone health. These exercises apply enough stress to bones to stimulate bone growth and density improvement, which is essential for combatting osteoporosis's effects. For instance, Seated Leg Presses against a resistance band can generate beneficial stress on the leg bones without the risks associated with high-impact exercises. Similarly, Seated BiCep Curls with light weights can strengthen the arm bones and muscles, supporting better overall bone health.

Balance and strength exercises are pivotal in reducing the risk of falls, a significant concern for individuals with osteoporosis. Falls can lead to fractures, particularly in a body with weakened bones. Therefore, Incorporating exercises that enhance balance and muscular strength is doubly beneficial. A seated toe tap, extending one leg and tapping the toe on the ground while maintaining an upright posture, can help improve balance and strengthen the leg muscles. Additionally, Seated Side Leg Raises, where you lift each leg to the side from a seated position, aid in maintaining the hip and core muscles, which are vital for good balance. Regular practice of these exercises can significantly mitigate the risk of falls by ensuring that the muscles involved in balance are stronger and more reactive.

The emphasis on maintaining correct posture during exercise must be balanced, especially for osteoporosis patients. Proper posture ensures that exercises are performed effectively and safely, minimizing stress on vulnerable bones and joints. Keeping the back straight and avoiding slouching is essential, which can put undue pressure on the spine and lead to discomfort or injury. A chair with good back support can help maintain proper alignment when performing any seated exercise. Additionally, being mindful of keeping your shoulders back and your abdomen engaged during exercises can reinforce good posture habits, which are beneficial during exercise and daily activities.

Consulting with healthcare professionals is invaluable for tailoring your exercise routine to suit osteoporosis-related needs. Each individual's condition can vary significantly in terms of severity and the presence of other health issues, making personalized advice crucial. To help design a program that maximizes benefits and minimizes risks, consult a physical therapist or a qualified fitness instructor who understands osteoporosis. They can recommend specific exercises that strengthen bones or improve balance based on your health status and bone density reports. Moreover, regular check-ups and consultations ensure that your exercise program evolves as your health needs change, providing ongoing support and guidance.

By incorporating these tailored exercise strategies into your routine, you can significantly improve your management of osteoporosis. Resistance training and weight-bearing exercises help maintain bone density and balance, and strength training reduces the risk of falls. Proper posture during exercises protects your bones, and professional guidance ensures your routine remains safe and effective. Together, these strategies form a comprehensive approach to staying active and healthy even with osteoporosis.

8.3 CARDIO ROUTINES FOR HEART HEALTH

The heart, a tireless engine, deserves attention and care, especially as it faces the natural challenges of aging. Designing cardiovascular exercises that boost heart health without overexertion is crucial. Low-impact cardio exercises are particularly beneficial as they increase your heart rate while minimizing stress on your body, making them ideal for seniors with existing heart conditions or those who are new to exercise. These exercises include Seated Marches or Arm Cycling, which can be performed comfortably in a chair. These gentle yet effective exercises encourage blood circulation and heart function without the jarring impact of more vigorous activities like running or jumping.

One effective routine involves Seated Rowing, where you pull towards yourself, mimicking the rowing motion, using a resistance band wrapped around a sturdy object. This gets your heart pumping and engages multiple muscle groups in a harmonious exercise that enhances cardiovascular endurance and muscular strength. Another beneficial activity is the Seated Overhead Press, which substitutes lightweight or canned goods. Lifting your arms above your head repeatedly increases your heart rate. It improves upper body strength, all while you are seated and stable.

Monitoring the intensity of your workouts is essential to ensure they are at a safe level for your heart. The perceived exertion scale, a user-friendly tool, helps you gauge the intensity of your exercise based on how hard you feel your body is working. The scale typically ranges from 1 (no exertion) to 10 (maximum effort). For most seniors, aiming for moderate exertion, around 3 to 4 on the scale, during cardio exercises is advisable. This range should have you breathing faster yet still able to carry on a conversation. Pairing this method with heart rate monitoring through a wearable device or manual pulse checks provides a comprehensive view of your exercise intensity, ensuring you stay within a heart-healthy range.

The frequency and duration of these activities are also vital factors in deriving cardiovascular benefits. According to guidelines from health organizations, seniors should engage in at least 150 minutes of moderate-intensity or 75 minutes of vigorous-intensity aerobic physical activity throughout the week. This can be broken down into manageable sessions, such as 30 minutes of low-impact cardio five times a week. Consistent, regular activity strengthens the heart muscle, helps manage weight, reduces stress levels, and improves overall energy.

Variety in your cardiovascular routine keeps the exercises engaging and effective. Alternating between chair-based cardio exercises can prevent boredom and ensure all muscle groups are involved over time, contributing to overall fitness and endurance. For instance, one day, you might focus on seated leg exercises. In contrast, you may concentrate on upper body movements on another day. Incorporating rhythmic activities like chair dancing once a week can also enhance your cardiovascular routine by introducing an enjoyable, socially engaging element to your workout, which can be incredibly uplifting and motivating.

This diverse approach to maintaining heart health through tailored, low-impact cardio exercises offers a pathway to enhanced well-being and vitality. By carefully monitoring exercise intensity and maintaining a regular schedule, you ensure these activities provide maximum benefit to your cardiovascular health without undue risk.

In wrapping up this chapter, we've explored how tailored exercises can significantly boost heart health and improve quality of life. These routines are designed to meet your fitness and capability level. This offers a safe and effective way to improve your physical health and, by extension, your independence. As we move forward, we continue to build on these foundations, exploring how chair exercises can be specifically adapted for those who use wheelchairs, ensuring everyone can engage in beneficial physical activity.

CHAIR EXERCISES FOR SENIORS SIMPLIFIED

THE ILLUSTRATED BEGINNER'S GUIDE TO IMPROVE YOUR BALANCE AND MOBILITY WITH EASY YOGA AND STRENGTH ROUTINES

"Helping one person might not change the world, but it could change the world for one person."

ANONYMOUS

As we get older, our bodies face new challenges, but staying active can make a big difference. Chair exercises are great because they are adaptable and help anyone improve their balance and mobility. This book is here to guide you through these exercises, making it easier to stay active and enjoy life.

Now, I have a small favor to ask you...

Would you help someone you've never met, even if you never got credit for it?

This person is just like you, or like you used to be—wanting to make a change, looking for guidance, and eager to live a healthier life. Our mission is to make "Chair Exercises for Seniors Simplified" available to everyone who needs it. But we need your help to reach more people.

Here's how you can help:

Please leave a review for this book.

Your review costs nothing and takes less than a minute, but it can make a huge difference. Your words could help...

...one more senior start a new exercise routine.
...one more grandparent play with their grandkids.
...one more friend take a stroll in the park.
...one more senior change their life for the better.
...one more dream come true.

To make this happen, you only need to leave a review. It's quick and easy!

Simply scan the QR code to leave your review:

If you feel good about helping another senior, you're my kind of person. Welcome to the club. You're one of us.

I'm excited to help you gain more strength and mobility with the exercises in this book. You'll love what's coming up in the following chapters.

Thank you from the bottom of my heart. Now, let's get back to improving your balance and mobility.

- Your biggest fan, Insight Editions

PS - Fun fact: When you help someone, you become more valuable to them. If you think this book can help another senior, please share it with them.

CHAPTER NINE

CHAIR EXERCISES FOR WHEELCHAIR USERS

9.1 UPPER BODY STRENGTH AND FLEXIBILITY FOR WHEELCHAIR USERS

Navigating life from a wheelchair shouldn't mean missing out on the profound benefits of physical exercise, particularly when it comes to strengthening and enhancing the flexibility of your upper body. These aspects are crucial for your general health and improving your daily functionality and independence. Regular upper body exercises can transform everyday tasks from daunting tasks into manageable, enjoyable routines.

Upper Body Conditioning: Strength exercises targeting the arms, shoulders, chest, and back to increase muscle tone and improve daily functioning

Building strength in your upper body involves a series of targeted exercises that engage your arms, shoulders, chest, and back. These exercises are pivotal as they compensate for lower body limitations by enhancing your ability to perform tasks such as pushing your wheelchair, lifting objects, and transferring yourself with ease. For instance, arm curls using lightweight dumbbells can significantly enhance bicep strength, which is essential for lifting or pulling movements. Similarly, shoulder presses, either with dumbbells or resistance bands, fortify your deltoids and triceps. These muscles are crucial for movements above your head and wheelchair propulsion.

To effectively increase muscle tone, consider incorporating resistance training into your routine. Resistance bands are instrumental as they are versatile and can be anchored to a door or a heavy piece of furniture, providing resistance when pulled. This training builds muscle and improves endurance, essential for wheelchair users who rely heavily on their upper body for mobility and daily activities.

Flexibility Focus: Stretching routines aimed at enhancing upper body flexibility, reducing the risk of muscle tightness and injury

Flexibility is equally important as strength, mainly to prevent the muscle tightness and joint stiffness that can develop from prolonged periods of sitting. Implementing a routine that includes stretches specifically designed for the shoulders, arms, and upper back can significantly reduce discomfort and enhance your range of motion. A simple yet effective stretch is the Arm Cross, where you gently pull one arm across your chest with the other, stretching the shoulder muscles. Another beneficial stretch is the Neck Tilt, which involves gently tilting your head toward each shoulder to stretch the neck muscles, relieving tension and maintaining neck flexibility.

Integrating these stretches into your daily routine is essential, ideally both at the beginning and end of your day. Consistent practice maintains flexibility and can significantly reduce injury risks due to sudden movements or extensive muscle strain.

Adaptive Equipment: Utilizing accessible equipment like resistance bands and lightweight dumbbells to add challenge to workouts

When selecting equipment for your workout, it's crucial to choose tools that enhance your exercise routine while accommodating your needs as a wheelchair user. Resistance bands are particularly beneficial due to their versatility and ease of use. Various exercises can be performed using them, thus targeting multiple muscle in the upper body. Their resistance can be easily adjusted by altering the length of the band or switching to bands of various thicknesses.

Lightweight dumbbells are another excellent choice, as they can be used for various exercises that build muscle strength and endurance. When starting with dumbbells, it's advisable to begin with a light weight and gradually increase as your strength improves, ensuring that you continue challenging your muscles without risking injury.

Engagement and Motivation: Encouraging consistent practice by integrating enjoyable activities and setting achievable goals

Staying motivated can often be the biggest challenge in maintaining a regular exercise regimen. To enhance engagement, try incorporating activities you enjoy into your exercise routine. For example, performing arm exercises in time with your favorite music can make the routine more enjoyable and less of a chore. Setting achievable and clear goals is also crucial for maintaining motivation. These goals range from being able to lift a certain weight, improving your flexibility enough to perform a specific task with ease, or simply committing to a set number of exercise sessions each week.

Consider integrating an interactive element such as a workout tracker or a journal where you can record your exercises, track your progress, and reflect on how your workouts impact your daily life. This helps keep you motivated by visually presenting your progress and allows you to adjust goals as you progress in your fitness journey.

Focusing on strengthening and flexibility exercises tailored to your needs as a wheelchair user, choosing the right equipment, and integrating enjoyable activities into your routine can significantly enhance your upper body conditioning. This improves your physical health and boosts your independence and quality of life, making everyday tasks more manageable and enjoyable.

9.2 CORE EXERCISES ADAPTED FOR WHEELCHAIR STABILITY

Strengthening your core is fundamental to enhancing your posture, balance, overall stability, and functionality in daily activities. For those using a wheelchair, core strength becomes even more vital, providing the necessary support to perform various tasks and movements efficiently. Regular core exercises can significantly improve your ability to maintain upright posture and confidently manage your mobility device.

Core stability exercises adaptable for wheelchair use are specially designed to target the muscles in your abdomen, lower back, and sides, which are crucial for maintaining good posture and balance. One effective exercise is the <u>Seated Abdominal Press</u>. This involves pressing your hands into your thighs while simultaneously contracting your abdominal muscles as if bracing for impact. This action strengthens the core muscles and teaches you how to activate your core during other activities, enhancing overall stability. Another beneficial exercise is the <u>Seated Oblique Twist</u>, where you hold onto your wheelchair's armrest with one hand and rotate your torso to the same side, while using your core muscles to control the movement. This exercise strengthens the sides of your abdomen. It improves your torso's rotational mobility, essential for tasks like reaching for objects to the side of your wheelchair.

Incorporating diaphragmatic breathing into your core exercises can dramatically enhance their effectiveness. This type of breathing involves fully engaging the diaphragm during inhalation, allowing the lungs to expand more fully. This, in turn, provides better oxygenation and aids in muscle performance. As you engage in a core exercise, focus on breathing deeply into your belly, feeling it expand and contract with every breath. This technique helps strengthen the core and promotes relaxation and stress reduction, making your exercise session more enjoyable and beneficial.

As you grow stronger, increasing the difficulty of your core exercises ensures continued progress and adaptation. You can achieve this by extending the duration of each exercise, adding more repetitions, or incorporating light weights or resistance bands for added resistance. For example, holding the abdominal press for a more extended period or performing more rotations during the oblique twists can make the exercises more challenging. Gradually increasing the difficulty of your workouts keeps your muscles engaged and growing and prevents the plateau effect, where progress can stall if the body becomes too accustomed to a certain level of activity.

Integrating core strengthening exercises into daily activities can significantly enhance their functionality and impact. For instance, consciously engaging your core while pushing your wheelchair or transferring from your wheelchair to another seat can transform these routine movements into opportunities for strengthening. Over time, these practices can substantially improve your core stability, making everyday tasks easier while also cutting down the risk of falls or injuries due to poor posture or weak core muscles.

Maintaining and enhancing your core strength is crucial to your overall health and mobility strategy. By focusing on core stability, incorporating effective breathing techniques, progressively challenging your muscles, and integrating core exercises into daily activities, you create a robust foundation for greater independence and a higher quality of life. These efforts ensure that your physical fitness regimen provides practical benefits that translate into real-world improvements, enabling you to navigate your daily life more easily and confidently.

As we conclude this chapter on specialized exercises for wheelchair users, we've explored how targeted upper body and core exercises can significantly enhance both your physical capabilities and your daily life. These exercises are designed to be integrated seamlessly into your routine, providing strength, flexibility, and stability that support various activities and tasks. Moving forward, we will delve into advanced chair exercise techniques, continuing to build on the foundation laid in this chapter further to enhance your strength, flexibility, and overall health.

CHAPTER TEN
ADVANCED CHAIR EXERCISE TECHNIQUES

As you continue to embrace chair exercises, enhancing your strength, flexibility, and overall well-being, there comes a time when you may feel ready to elevate your routine. Advanced chair exercise techniques allow you to deepen your practice, challenge your body in new ways, and see even more significant improvements in your health and mobility. This chapter has been designed to guide you through safely increasing the intensity of your exercises, to ensure you continue to make improvements without risking injury or exhaustion.

10.1 INCREASING EXERCISE INTENSITY SAFELY

Intensity Indicators: Understanding How to Gauge Exercise Intensity and Recognize When It's Safe to Progress to More Challenging Movements

Knowing when and how to increase your workout intensity safely is crucial to avoid overexertion while continuing to benefit from your exercise regimen. One fundamental way to gauge the intensity of your exercises is to monitor your heart rate and breathing. It would help if you aimed to reach a level where your breath quickens, but you are not so out of breath that you can't hold a conversation. This is often called the "talk test" and is a reliable, real-time indicator of your exercise intensity.

Additionally, paying attention to how your muscles feel during and after workouts can provide insights into whether you work within an appropriate intensity range. While it's normal to feel some muscle fatigue, you should not experience sharp pain or discomfort that lasts more than a couple of hours post-exercise. This could indicate that you've pushed too hard and must adjust your intensity.

Advanced Modifications: Techniques for Adding Complexity to Existing Exercises, Such as Increased Repetitions, Longer Holds, or Added Resistance

Once you're comfortable with the basics and can perform exercises without undue fatigue or discomfort, consider incorporating advanced modifications to enhance their difficulty and effectiveness. For instance, if you've been performing seated leg lifts, you might increase the number of repetitions or add a brief hold at the top of the lift to challenge your muscles further. Similarly, incorporating resistance bands or light weights can significantly increase the intensity of arm exercises, such as bicep curls or shoulder presses.

Advanced modifications make the exercises more challenging and help prevent the plateau effect, where improvements in strength and endurance slow down or stall. Continuously adapting and intensifying your workouts ensures ongoing progress and sustained interest in your exercise routine.

Listening to Your Body: Emphasizing the Importance of Paying Attention to the Body's Signals to Avoid Overexertion and Injury

Listening to your body becomes even more critical as you advance in your exercise routine. Recognizing the difference between the everyday physical challenge of a more intense workout and signs that you may be pushing too hard is essential. Symptoms like dizziness, unusual or sharp pain, and extreme fatigue indicate that you need to scale back and possibly consult a healthcare provider.

Maintaining a balanced approach to your workouts is vital. It's tempting to push through discomfort, hoping for faster gains, but respecting your body's limits is essential for long-term health and fitness.

Recovery and Rest: The Crucial Role of Rest and Recovery in an Advanced Exercise Routine, Ensuring Muscles Have Time to Repair and Strengthen

Rest and recovery are foundational elements of any advanced exercise routine. After challenging your muscles with more intense or complex exercises, giving them time to repair and strengthen is vital. This helps prevent injury and is crucial for muscle growth and overall fitness improvement.

Incorporating days of lighter activity or complete rest into your exercise schedule allows your body to recover and adapt to the increased demands you've placed on it. During rest periods, processes that stimulate muscle repair and growth are activated, and your body replenishes energy stores and rebuilds damaged tissues. This is not a sign of slacking off but a critical part of an advanced fitness regimen.

Interactive Element: Reflective Journaling Prompt

Consider keeping a reflective exercise journal to help you monitor your progress and the effects of increasing exercise intensity after each workout; jot down what exercises you did, any modifications you made, how you felt during and after the exercises, and any signs of overexertion you might have experienced. Reflecting on this journal can help you fine-tune your routine, making necessary adjustments to continue safely challenging yourself without risking your health. This practice keeps you engaged with your fitness goals and cultivates a deeper connection with your body's needs and responses.

Embracing these advanced techniques in chair exercise allows you to continue your progress toward more excellent health and vitality. By carefully monitoring exercise intensity, incorporating advanced modifications, listening to your body, and prioritizing recovery, you set the stage for sustained success in your fitness journey. As you implement these strategies, remember that each step forward, no matter how small, is a significant stride towards a healthier, more vibrant you.

10.2 COMBINING MOVEMENTS FOR COMPOUND WORKOUTS

Compound exercises involving multiple muscle groups engaged simultaneously, which is a game-changer in fitness, particularly for chair-based routines. These exercises offer a streamlined approach to working out, allowing you to achieve comprehensive strength and flexibility benefits in a shorter period. The efficiency of compound movements lies in their ability to simulate daily activities that require the coordination of several muscle groups, thus enhancing muscular strength and functional fitness.

Let's delve deeper into why compound movements are so beneficial. When you perform an exercise that recruits multiple muscle groups, such as a seated row that engages both the arms and the back, you save time and increase the caloric expenditure compared to isolated exercises. This integrated approach to muscle engagement mirrors how your body naturally operates, making compound exercises particularly effective for enhancing your ability to perform everyday tasks. Additionally, these exercises can improve intermuscular coordination and excellent core stability, as your core often supports and stabilizes your body during these movements.

Designing compound exercise routines requires thoughtful consideration to ensure balance and effectiveness. When creating a compound workout schedule, aim to include movements that work opposite muscle groups, which helps prevent muscle imbalances and provides a harmonious development of strength. For instance, if one exercise focuses on the muscles in the front of the body, like the chest and quadriceps, the next should involve the muscles in the back, such as the hamstrings and upper back. This approach keeps the workout balanced and maximizes your time by engaging the whole body across a series of exercises.

Let's explore some examples of compound exercises suitable for chair routines, providing step-by-step instructions to ensure proper form and effectiveness. A great example is the seated chest press combined with a leg extension. Start by sitting securely in your chair with your back straight. Hold weights in both hands at chest level, and as you press the weights forward, simultaneously extend one leg straight out. This movement engages your chest, shoulders, triceps, and quadriceps, offering a robust workout. Return to the starting position and repeat, alternating the leg you extend with each repetition. This exercise strengthens multiple muscle groups and challenges your coordination and balance, enhancing overall body functionality.

Adapting these compound movements to fit your fitness level and mobility is crucial to making the exercises both achievable and challenging. It is essential to start at a level that feels doable for you, which might mean using lighter weights or performing fewer repetitions as you begin. Your strength and flexibility will improve over time, as you increase the complexity of the movements by adding more weight, additional repetitions, or incorporating slightly more challenging versions of the exercises. For example, suppose the seated chest press with leg extension becomes too comfortable. In that case, add a slight twist to your torso with each press, engaging the core muscles more intensively.

By integrating compound movements into your chair exercise routine, you enhance the efficiency and effectiveness of your workouts, enabling significant improvements in your strength, flexibility, and overall functional fitness. These exercises provide a comprehensive approach to maintaining and enhancing physical health, making everyday activities more manageable and enjoyable.While you continue to adapt and evolve your routine, remember that each new challenge brings an opportunity for growth and improvement, reinforcing the benefits of your commitment to staying active and healthy.

10.3 INTEGRATING SMALL WEIGHTS FOR ADDED RESISTANCE

The simple addition of small weights to your chair exercise routine can significantly amplify the benefits of your workouts. By incorporating this resistance element, you're not merely moving; you're genuinely challenging your muscles to strengthen and endure more, enhancing your overall strength and stamina. This evolution in your exercise regimen is essential for continuing to see improvements in your physical health as you adapt to previous workouts.

The benefits of adding small weights are manifold. Resistance training while lifting small hand weights can lead to greater muscle strength, crucial for maintaining mobility and independence. It also enhances muscle endurance, allowing you to perform daily activities, like carrying groceries or standing up from a chair, with greater ease and less fatigue. Furthermore, this training can contribute to better bone health, which is particularly important for seniors to help against the natural decline in bone density that comes with age.

When starting with weights, selecting the appropriate weight is crucial to ensure safety and effectiveness. It's advisable to begin with light weights that do not strain your muscles or joints but are still challenging enough to improve your strength. A good rule of thumb is to choose a weight with which you can perform about 12 to 15 repetitions of an exercise; the last few repetitions should feel challenging but still doable. While your strength improves, you can gradually increase your weight, ensuring continuous improvement and adaptation in your workout regimen.

Incorporating these weights into your chair exercises requires careful attention to form and technique to avoid injury. For example, when performing a Seated Shoulder Press, hold the weights at shoulder height with your elbows bent and palms facing forward. As you press the weights upward, extend your arms completely but do not lock your elbows, then slowly lower them back to the starting position. Ensuring that movements are controlled and steady not only maximizes the effectiveness of the exercise but also minimizes the risk of straining muscles or joints.

Monitoring your progress as you integrate weights into your regimen is essential for motivation and safety. Regularly assess how the exercises feel—whether they continue to be challenging or have become too easy. If you find the exercises less demanding, it may be time to increase the weight slightly. Conversely, if you experience discomfort or undue fatigue, reducing the weight or revisiting your technique may be necessary. Keeping a simple log of the weights you use, the exercises you perform, and your responses to them can help you track your progress and make informed adjustments over time.

As you integrate small weights into your chair exercises, you'll discover that this slight modification can profoundly transform your workout routine, providing new challenges and renewed bene-fits. This advancement in your exercise regimen shows your commitment to maintaining and enhancing your physical health and independence.

In wrapping up this exploration of advanced chair exercise tech-niques, we've delved into the strategic integration of increased intensity, compound movements, and added resistance to enrich your workouts. These enhancements are designed to maintain and elevate your fitness level, ensuring continued improvement and adaptation. As you continue to embrace these advanced techniques, remember that each new challenge offers growth and more excel-lent well-being opportunities. As the journey continues, we will explore how to maintain motivation and consistency in your exer-cise routine, which are essential components for long-term success and enjoyment in your fitness journey.

CHAPTER ELEVEN
PAIN MANAGEMENT AND INJURY PREVENTION

A s we age, our bodies tell stories in whispers and occasional shouts, reminding us of the long roads we've traveled. Engaging in physical activity like chair exercises can increase the volume of these bodily signals, making it crucial to discern what your body is communicating. This chapter will explore the nuances between good pain, which signals growth, and bad pain, which might indicate potential harm or injury. This distinction is pivotal in maintaining a healthy, active lifestyle that respects your body's limits and capabilities.

11.1 LISTENING TO YOUR BODY: RECOGNIZING GOOD PAIN VS. BAD PAIN

Understanding Pain Signals: Differentiating between the discomfort that indicates a beneficial workout and pain that may signal injury or overexertion

When you begin to exercise, encountering discomfort is a natural part of the process. This type of pain, often referred to as "good pain," manifests as a mild burn or fatigue in muscles during or shortly after your workout. It's a sign that your muscles are being pushed slightly beyond their usual limits, essential for growth and strengthening. This sensation should not be sharp or debilitating. Still, it should feel more like a stretch or a strain that decreases as your body gets accustomed to the exercise. Your body adapts to new challenges, leading to greater endurance and strength.

On the other hand, "bad pain" can feel sharp and stabbing or cause discomfort that persists long after exercising. It can occur during an exercise or might appear as delayed pain, indicating that something isn't right, such as a strain, sprain, or worse, an injury that needs attention. This type of pain might be localized to a joint or a specific part of your body, signaling that you've potentially overexerted or performed an exercise incorrectly.

Responding to Pain: Appropriate responses to various types of pain, including when to rest, modify exercises, or seek medical attention

When encountering good pain, the best response is to allow your body a brief rest period. This doesn't necessarily mean stopping all activity. Rather, minimize the intensity level or how often you exercise to allow muscles to recover. Hydrating and performing gentle stretches can also facilitate muscle recovery and ease discomfort.

If you experience bad pain, you should immediately stop the exercise that caused it to prevent further harm. Applying cold packs can help reduce immediate inflammation, followed by gentle heat after 24 hours to promote blood flow and healing. Adjusting the exercise to help minimize stress on the affected area is crucial if the pain persists despite these measures. For instance, if a particular movement causes knee pain, switching to exercises focusing more on upper body strength can help maintain your activity levels safely.

If adjustments and rest do not alleviate the pain, or if the pain is severe and limits mobility, you must contact your healthcare provider. They will diagnose your condition and provide safe and effective instructions or treatment options, ensuring your exercise routine does not compromise your health.

Chronic vs. Acute Pain: Discussing the characteristics of chronic and acute pain and how exercise routines can be adjusted to accommodate each

Chronic pain can be persistent and lasts days, weeks, or even longer. It is often unrelated to an acute injury. It can be due to ongoing arthritis or other musculoskeletal issues. Managing chronic pain involves regular, moderate exercise that maintains mobility without exacerbating the pain. Chair exercises can be particularly beneficial as they can be easily adapted to minimize discomfort while providing physical benefits.

Acute pain, however, occurs suddenly and is usually sharp and severe. It typically signals an injury or a condition that urgently needs addressing. In such cases, it's critical to pause your exercise routine and seek medical evaluation to understand the underlying cause of the pain.

Pain Management Techniques: Introducing non-pharmacological pain management techniques suitable for seniors, such as heat/cold therapy, massage, and relaxation exercises

Managing pain effectively often requires a combination of methods tailored to your needs and conditions. Non-pharmacological techniques are particularly appealing as they have fewer side effects than medication. Heat therapy can be helpful for chronic pain, such as that caused by arthritis, as it helps relax and soothe stiff joints and muscles, improving mobility. Conversely, cold therapy is best for acute injuries or pain, reducing inflammation and numbing sore tissues.

Massage is another effective way to manage pain, particularly chronic pain, by improving circulation and muscle function, which can alleviate stiffness and discomfort. Gentle, regular massages can also promote relaxation and well-being, which in itself can help manage pain better.

Relaxation exercises, including deep breathing, mindfulness, and gentle yoga, can also significantly affect pain management. These techniques help reduce overall stress and tension, which can exacerbate pain perceptions, providing a sense of control and well-being that can make pain more manageable.

Pain management techniques can be incorporated into your routine. They can provide you with an arsenal of tools to tackle pain effectively, ensuring that it does not deter you from leading an active, fulfilling life. As you continue engaging with these practices, remember that understanding and listening to your body's signals is vital in maintaining a balanced, health-conscious exercise and pain management approach.

11.2 WARM-UP AND COOL-DOWN: ESSENTIAL FOR INJURY PREVENTION

Understanding the importance of a proper warm-up must be balanced to keep our bodies healthy and limber in later years. Initiating any physical activity with a warm-up is a gentle invitation for your body to prepare for more vigorous activity. It's akin to turning the key in your car's ignition on a cold day; you're essentially preparing the engine to perform optimally. Similarly, gradually increasing your heart rate and loosening your muscles through specific movements significantly reduce the risk of straining muscles or stressing joints, which can lead to injuries. For seniors especially, where muscles and joints might be more susceptible to injury, a thorough warm-up can be the difference between a beneficial exercise session and one that ends in discomfort.

A tailored warm-up routine should target the muscle groups engaged during your main exercise session, particularly one that can be performed in a chair. This ensures that these muscles are warmed and more elastic, ready to handle the upcoming exertions. For instance, if your exercise session involves upper body movements, your warm-up could include arm circles, shoulder shrugs, and gentle twists of your torso. Each movement should be performed slowly and focused on breathing deeply to increase oxygen flow to your muscles. Starting with small movements, gradually increase the range of motion as your body feels looser. This prepares your muscles and syncs your mind with your body, helping you focus on the activity.

The value of a proper cool-down phase mirrors that of the warm-up, yet it serves a different purpose. After engaging in physical activity, your body needs a transition period to return to its resting state. Please do not skip this step, as it builds lactic acid in your muscles, often contributing to post-exercise soreness. Additionally, an abrupt cessation of activity can cause your heart rate and blood pressure to drop precipitously, which might lead to dizziness or feelings of light-headedness. By doing a cool-down, you gradually slow your heart rate and stretch out the muscles that have been exerted, aiding in recovery and reducing the likelihood of stiffness later on.

Practical cool-down exercises often involve gentle stretching and relaxation techniques that help lengthen and relax your muscles and give you a moment to reflect on the workout you've completed. For instance, following a session with a lot of leg work, you might perform seated hamstring stretches or ankle rolls. Each stretch should be held for 15 to 30 seconds, allowing your muscles to relax gradually. Breathing also plays a crucial role here; with each exhale, try to deepen the stretch slightly, promoting flexibility and helping to flush out any remaining muscle tension.

Incorporating these mindful practices of warming up and cooling down into your regular exercise routine maximizes the benefits of physical activity. It shows a deep respect for your body's capabilities and limits. By preparing your body adequately before exercise and helping it recover afterward, you are investing in your health and ensuring you can enjoy an active, fulfilling lifestyle.

11.3 ADDRESSING COMMON EXERCISE-RELATED ACHES

Navigating through the aches accompanying physical activities is almost a rite of passage as we age. However, understanding these discomforts can transform them from deterrents to guides that help optimize our exercise routines. Most seniors will experience some form of post-exercise ache due to the natural aging process, which often involves the weakening of muscles and less fluid joints. Recognizing the everyday aches—like muscle soreness or mild joint pain after a new or intensified routine—is crucial. Typically, these aches are a natural response to the microscopic tears in muscle fibers during exercise. This is part of how muscles rebuild stronger. Still, it's essential to differentiate between these expected sensations and symptoms that may indicate something more serious, such as sharp, stabbing pains or pain that doesn't subside with rest and appropriate aftercare.

Muscle soreness that appears a day or two after exercising often called delayed-onset muscle soreness (DOMS), is a normal response to physical activity that challenges the muscle beyond its usual level. It's a sign that your muscles are adapting, growing stronger in response to the demands placed on them. However, joint pains or aches that persist could indicate an overuse injury or inflammation, and these should not be dismissed as they could lead to more severe injuries or chronic issues if not appropriately addressed.

Addressing these everyday aches effectively begins with basic first aid measures, which can often be managed at home. For instance, the RICE method—rest, ice, compression, and elevation—is particularly effective for managing minor strains or joint discomfort. Rest is vital as it allows the affected tissues to recover and prevents further strain. Ice packs applied in intervals can help reduce swelling and soothe pain. Reduce swelling and provide support by adding compression with an elastic bandage. At the same time, the elevation of the injured part above the heart level can further help reduce swelling by draining excess fluid.

Moving on to when professional help might be necessary, it's vital to be vigilant and responsive to what your body is telling you. If the pain is severe, limits mobility, significantly changes character, or doesn't improve with primary home care, these could be red flags signaling the need for a medical evaluation. Persistent pain might indicate underlying conditions such as arthritis flare-ups or fractures, especially if the pain is localized and sharp. Professional evaluations ensure that appropriate treatments can be administered and serious complications are avoided.

Lastly, injury prevention should be the cornerstone of any exercise regimen, especially for seniors. This is not only about handling injuries after they occur but also about implementing strategies to prevent them. Listening to your body is paramount; understanding and respecting your body's limits daily can guide your exercise intensity and avoid overexertion. Employing correct exercise techniques is equally crucial. You must comprehend the proper form for each exercise to minimize the chance of injuries caused by incorrect posture or movements.

Moreover, integrating rest days into your exercise routine is essential. These days are not about inactivity but about allowing your body to recover and strengthen. Regular, moderate exercise interspersed with adequate rest prevents the cycle of overuse and injury, supporting a sustainable and beneficial exercise habit.

In conclusion, addressing everyday exercise-related aches involves:

- A balanced approach to recognizing normal post-exercise discomforts.
- Employing effective first aid.
- Knowing when to seek professional advice.
- Preventing injuries through mindful exercise practices.

As we move forward, remember that each step taken in understanding and responding to your body's signals is a step towards maintaining a healthy, active lifestyle that supports your independence and well-being. Looking ahead, we will explore the nutritional aspects of maintaining an active lifestyle, focusing on how the right foods can help your exercise goals and overall health.

CHAPTER TWELVE

NUTRITION AND HYDRATION

I magine your body as a beautifully intricate machine. Just like any high-performance mechanism, the quality of fuel you put into it significantly affects how well it functions. For us, this fuel is the food and drinks we consume. Navigating through the golden years, the impact of nutrition takes on an even greater importance. It's not just about eating to quell hunger—it's about nourishing your body to support strength, vitality, and recovery, especially when paired with your exercise routine. In the following chapter, we'll explore how a customized and nutritionally balanced diet can improve the quality of life for seniors and support their physical activities.

12.1 EATING FOR STRENGTH: NUTRITIONAL GUIDELINES FOR SENIORS

Balanced Diet Principles

A balanced diet is foundational to maintaining health and enhancing the quality of life as you age. It's about ensuring your meals are rich in essential nutrients catering to senior-specific health needs. Proteins, for instance, are crucial for muscle maintenance and repair. As we get older, our bodies tend to experience a loss of muscle mass, often called sarcopenia. Including adequate high-quality protein sources like lean meats, fish, eggs, and legumes can help mitigate this loss, preserving muscle strength and function, which is vital for everyday activities.

Calcium and vitamin D are non-negotiables for maintaining healthy bones. With age, bones can become more fragile, making you susceptible to fractures. Various dairy products like cheese, milk, and yogurt are excellent calcium sources, an essential nutrient for the body. In contrast, vitamin D, crucial for calcium absorption, can be sourced from sunlight exposure, fatty fish, and fortified foods. Including various fruits and vegetables in your daily meals can benefit your body, as they contain abundant vitamins and minerals that help maintain cellular well-being and boost the immune system.

Meal Planning and Preparation

Planning and preparing meals might seem daunting, primarily if you're catering to specific dietary needs or managing decreased appetite, which is common among seniors. However, simple strategies can make this process enjoyable and ensure you eat nutritiously. Start planning your meals weekly. This helps you shop for the right ingredients and provides a variety of nutrients in your diet. Prepare dishes that are easy to cook yet flavorful, like stews, casseroles, or salads packed with nuts and seeds for added nutrition. For those with dietary restrictions, such as low sodium for heart health or gluten-free for celiac disease, focus on natural, whole foods like vegetables, fruits, lean proteins, and whole grains that naturally meet these criteria.

Supplementation Considerations

While a balanced diet is ideal, specific nutritional needs might not be fully met through diet alone, especially in seniors. Common deficiencies, such as vitamin D, vitamin B12, and calcium, may need to be addressed with supplements. For example, vitamin B12 is essential for nerve function, DNA, and red blood cell production, but its absorption decreases as we age. It is vital to consult with a healthcare provider before taking any supplements to discuss your specific needs based on your diet, lifestyle, and medical conditions.

Nutrition and Exercise Synergy

"The effectiveness of your exercise routine can be significantly influenced by the food you eat." Proper nutrition supports energy levels, aids recovery, and enhances overall performance. Carbohydrates are essential for energy, so including moderate amounts of whole grains or starchy vegetables in your meals can help fuel your exercise sessions. After exercising, consuming proteins and some carbohydrates is essential to aid muscle recovery and replenish energy stores. This synergy between diet and exercise is crucial for maintaining an active and healthy lifestyle, ensuring you reap the maximum benefits from your fitness efforts.

By focusing on these critical aspects of nutrition, you equip your body with the best resources to support an active lifestyle, enhance your strength and mobility, and ensure a more prosperous, vibrant senior life. As we continue exploring how proper hydration complements this nutritional framework, remember that each meal is an opportunity to nourish your body and your zest for life.

12.2 STAYING HYDRATED: THE ROLE OF WATER IN SENIOR HEALTH

Understanding the pivotal role of hydration in maintaining health is akin to appreciating the necessity of oil in keeping a machine running smoothly. Water is crucial to various bodily functions, including regulating body temperature, transporting nutrients, and eliminating wastes. For seniors, staying adequately hydrated is even more critical due to physiological changes that come with aging, which can alter the body's fluid balance and sometimes blunt the sensation of thirst.

Hydration is essential for maintaining all cells' health and proper circulation, digestion, and kidney function. However, dehydration is a common issue among seniors, often because the sense of thirst diminishes with age. Dehydration can have serious consequences, impacting everything from renal function to cognitive ability. It can exacerbate chronic conditions such as kidney stones and urinary tract infections. It can also lead to more acute, severe conditions like heat stroke. Therefore, understanding and recognizing the signs of dehydration is crucial. These signs can be subtle, ranging from dry mouth, fatigue, and dizziness to more severe symptoms such as rapid heartbeat, low blood pressure, and confusion.

For proper hydration, it's advisable to adopt proactive hydration strategies. One effective method is to integrate the habit of drinking fluids regularly throughout the day rather than waiting to feel thirsty. Setting reminders regularly through a smartphone app or a simple timer can be an excellent way to ensure consistent fluid intake. Incorporating food items with high water content in your diet can assist you in maintaining proper hydration levels and enhance overall hydration. Fruits like watermelon, strawberries, oranges, and vegetables like cucumbers, lettuce, and celery provide nutrients and contribute to your overall fluid intake.

Hydration plays a crucial role in physical activity, especially for seniors engaging in exercise routines like chair exercises. Ensuring you are well-hydrated before starting your workout can prevent premature fatigue and help maintain optimal muscle function. Keeping a water bottle within reach during training can encourage regular sips between routines. At the same time, post-exercise hydration is vital to recovery and helps replenish fluids lost through sweat. This practice supports recovery and prepares your body for subsequent physical activities, maintaining a cycle of health and activity that fosters overall well-being.

By adopting these hydration practices, you ensure that your body has the necessary resources to perform at its best, supporting your active lifestyle and contributing to your overall health management. As we progress, remember that each sip of water is a step towards maintaining vitality and enhancing your capacity to enjoy daily activities. This focus on hydration, combined with the nutritional strategies discussed earlier, forms a comprehensive approach to wellness that empowers you to lead a healthier, more fulfilled life.

In wrapping up this chapter on nutrition and hydration, we've discussed essential dietary principles and practical hydration strategies that fortify your body's health. By incorporating nutritional and hydration insights, you can improve the effectiveness of your physical activities and better understand how closely intertwined they are with your overall health and wellness. As we progress, the journey continues, focusing on the importance of sleep in recovery and overall health, further building our foundation for maintaining vitality and enhancing quality of life.

CHAPTER THIRTEEN

THE ROLE OF SLEEP IN RECOVERY

T hink of sleep as a team of silent renovators who work diligently to repair the damage caused by our daily routine as we rest. For seniors, this nightly restoration is beneficial and crucial for maintaining a vibrant, active lifestyle. As we delve into the significant influence of sleep on our health and recovery, you'll learn accessible practices to improve the quality of your sleep. Additionally, you'll learn how incorporating chair exercises into your daily routine can improve sleep, ultimately promoting overall well-being.

13.1 OPTIMIZING YOUR SLEEP FOR BETTER HEALTH

Sleep and Health Connection

The link between good sleep and health is well-documented yet often underestimated, especially as we age. Quality sleep is pivotal in muscle recovery, immune function, and overall well-being. During sleep, the body undergoes various processes that repair muscle tissue and restore energy. This is crucial for seniors who engage in physical activities such as chair exercises, as adequate rest is needed to reap the full benefits of exercise without risking injury.

Moreover, sleep significantly affects immune function. Studies have shown that well-rested individuals have a more robust immune response, vital for fighting infections and maintaining health. This is particularly important for seniors, as the immune system naturally weakens with age. Additionally, sleep impacts many other areas of health, including cognitive function and emotional stability, making it a cornerstone of a healthy lifestyle.

Sleep Needs for Seniors

As we get older, there are changes in our sleep patterns. Seniors may notice a difference in their circadian rhythms, determining when they sleep and wake up. This can result in going to bed earlier and waking up earlier. However, it's important to note that the amount of sleep needed remains the same with age. Seniors typically need around 7 to 8 hours of sleep per night. Sleep quality and quantity are both equally important to a restful night. Achieving deep sleep stages is crucial because these are the periods when the body performs most of its healing and therapeutic functions.

Improving Sleep Quality

Having better quality sleep can bring about a remarkable change in your life. There are a few techniques that you can use to achieve this. One such method is setting up a regular sleep schedule, which can help synchronize your internal clock to make it simpler to fall asleep and awake naturally. Creating a bedtime routine can signal your body that it's time to wind down. This routine might include reading a book, listening to soft music, or doing gentle stretches, which can be particularly beneficial for relaxing the muscles and preparing your body for sleep.

Managing sleep disturbances is also crucial. Nighttime awakenings or restless leg syndrome can significantly impact sleep quality for many seniors. Addressing these disturbances might involve dietary adjustments, such as reducing fluid intake before bed to minimize nighttime trips to the bathroom or consulting a healthcare provider for conditions like sleep apnea or restless leg syndrome.

Exercise's Role in Sleep

Regular physical activity, including chair exercises, has dramatically improved sleep quality. Exercise promotes more extended periods of deep sleep, which are crucial for physical health and cognitive function. However, timing is vital. Participating in mentally stimulating activities right before bedtime can adversely impact it by making it difficult to fall asleep. Try to schedule your exercise sessions for earlier in the day. Morning routines are particularly effective as they help reinforce the natural circadian rhythm, promoting daytime alertness and nighttime sleepiness.

Visual Element: Sleep and Exercise Tracker

Consider maintaining a sleep and exercise tracker to help you monitor the relationship between your exercise habits and sleep quality. This tool can be a simple chart that logs your daily exercise routine, the times you go to bed and wake up, and a rating for your sleep quality each night. Over time, this visual record can offer valuable insights into how your physical activity impacts your sleep patterns, allowing you to make informed adjustments for better health outcomes.

In exploring these aspects of sleep and its critical role in recovery, the goal is to provide you with the knowledge and tools necessary to enhance your sleep quality. By prioritizing your physical well-being, you can improve your overall life quality and approach your senior years with vigor and fortitude, enabling you to make the most of this stage of life. As we delve into the intricate relationship between sleep and recovery, remember that every night offers an opportunity for renewal and restoration, essential for thriving in your daily activities and maintaining your independence.

13.2 CREATING A RESTFUL ENVIRONMENT: TIPS FOR SENIORS

Setting the right environment for a good night's sleep is like creating a peaceful and refreshing haven every evening. Your bedroom should be a tranquil sanctuary that encourages relaxation and comfort, which is vital for achieving rejuvenating and restful sleep. To achieve this, consider the sensory experiences of your bedroom: the lighting, noise, and temperature all play critical roles in influencing sleep quality. Soft, dimmable lights can help signal to your body that it's time to wind down, while blackout curtains or shades can block out intrusive street lights or early morning sunlight. Noise can significantly disrupt sleep; therefore, minimizing it is crucial. You might use a white noise machine or earplugs to drown out ambient sounds. Keeping your bedroom at a relaxed, comfortable temperature, generally between 60 and 67 degrees Fahrenheit, also facilitates better sleep, as cooler temperatures signal to your body that it's time to sleep.

The physical support provided by your mattress and pillows is equally vital. Suppose your mattress doesn't provide adequate support. In that case, it can result in discomfort and pain, particularly for those with pre-existing conditions like back problems or arthritis. Investing in a high-quality mattress that provides comfort and support according to your body's needs is worthwhile. It's often helpful to test different types of mattresses in-store to find one that suits your comfort preferences.

Similarly, the right pillow can make a substantial difference. Pillows need to uphold the natural curve of your neck. Orthopedic pillows may help with chronic neck or back pain. Replacing your mattress and pillows every few years helps maintain their support.

In today's fast-paced world, it's easy to carry the stimulation of the day right up to bedtime, but doing so can significantly impair your ability to fall asleep. Limiting the intake of stimulants such as caffeine and nicotine in the hours before bedtime is crucial as they can keep you awake. It is essential to restrict the use of smartphones, tablets, and televisions, especially before bed. Specific electronic devices like smartphones and laptops emit blue light that can disrupt melatonin production, a hormone responsible for regulating sleep. To improve overall sleep quality, avoiding these devices for at least an hour before bedtime is recommended. Instead, you can read a book or listen to calming music, which can help signal your brain that it's time to wind down.

Adding relaxation techniques to your evening routine can increase your ability to fall asleep and have a restful night. Techniques such as gentle stretching can relieve physical tension and help prepare your body for rest. Stretching your arms, legs, and back gently can be particularly soothing. Engaging in deep breathing exercises effectively clears your mind of the clutter from a busy day. Encouraging your body to relax by taking slow, deep breaths can help you fall asleep more easily. Meditation, too, can be a powerful tool for calming the mind and easing into sleep. Several guided meditations are specifically designed to promote sleep, focusing on relaxing imagery or calming sounds that help you drift off to sleep.

By combining these strategies, you can take a comprehensive approach to getting a good night's sleep. By optimizing your bedroom environment, moderating stimulant intake, and engaging in relaxation practices, you set the stage for deep, restorative sleep that supports your overall health and well-being.

As this chapter closes, remember that sleep is not merely a pause in your day but a critical component of your health regimen, as vital as nutrition and exercise. Each element discussed here—from the tranquility of your bedroom setting to the rituals that ready your mind and body for rest—works synergistically to enhance your sleep quality. The following section will explore how maintaining an active lifestyle can improve mental and emotional well-being. Additionally, we will establish a connection between physical activity, restful sleep, and overall holistic health. By taking a comprehensive approach, you can ensure that you receive complete support in your endeavors to live a fulfilling and vibrant life in your senior years.

CHAPTER FOURTEEN

THE MENTAL AND EMOTIONAL BENEFITS OF CHAIR EXERCISES

I magine a world where every movement you make sends waves of positivity through your mind and body, where each stretch and bend strengthens your muscles and unwinds your thoughts and emotions. This world isn't far-fetched—it's accessible here and now through chair exercises. These activities are not only about maintaining physical health; they are profoundly potent tools for enhancing mental and emotional well-being.

14.1 EXERCISE AS STRESS RELIEF: THE PSYCHOLOGICAL UPSIDES

Endorphin Release: The Natural Mood Enhancer

When you engage in chair exercises, your body does more than move; it also chemically enhances your mood. These movements stimulate the release of endorphins, often known as the body's "feel-good" hormones. Endorphins are natural stress fighters; they combat feelings of stress and pain by triggering a positive feeling in the body that is similar to that of morphine. For you, this means that every session of chair exercises not only helps you stay fit but also naturally elevates your mood and creates a sense of well-being. This biochemical change is particularly beneficial as it provides a healthy, drug-free method to manage and reduce stress and anxiety, making it an invaluable tool for your emotional health toolkit.

Mindfulness in Motion: Enhancing Mental Clarity and Emotional Tranquility

Chair exercises also offer a unique opportunity to practice mindfulness. Mindfulness involves remaining entirely focused and aware of our thoughts, emotions, physical sensations, and the environment surrounding us at every moment. When you perform a seated stretch or a muscle-strengthening exercise, you can focus intently on your breath, the movement of your muscles, and how they feel, which helps anchor you in the present moment. Being present can significantly reduce the chatter of daily worries and stresses, clarify your thoughts, and bring about a peaceful state of mind. Incorporating mindfulness into your exercise regimen can elevate it from merely a physical activity to a meditative practice. This can enhance the emotional advantages and help you attain a more tranquil and centered state of mind.

Routine and Structure: Bringing Order to Daily Life

Integrating a regular schedule of chair exercises into your daily life introduces structure and routine, which can be incredibly stabilizing. Routine helps reduce anxiety by providing predictability—a comfort in knowing what will happen next, making the world feel less chaotic. For seniors, who often face multiple changes from health to lifestyle, having a structured exercise routine can provide a sense of normalcy and control. This predictability helps manage mental health, reduce feelings of helplessness and stress, and improve overall mood stability.

Coping Mechanism: A Healthy Outlet for Stress and Negative Emotions

Lastly, chair exercises are a healthy coping mechanism for managing stress and negative emotions. Instead of turning to potentially harmful coping strategies such as overeating, smoking, or inactivity, chair exercises provide a productive and beneficial outlet. They offer a way to channel your energy and frustrations into movement, which can help clear your mind and reduce feelings of depression or anxiety. Furthermore, physical activity can be a distraction, allowing you to take a break from the stressors that occupy your thoughts, which can be especially helpful in processing emotions more effectively.

Chair exercises can contribute to your overall health as you age by improving your physical health and strengthening your mental and emotional resilience. Therefore, they play a vital role in a holistic approach to wellness. As you continue to embrace these exercises, you gradually cultivate a more robust, serene, and balanced lifestyle, reflecting the profound interconnectedness of mind and body.

14.2 BUILDING CONFIDENCE AND INDEPENDENCE THROUGH MOVEMENT

Mastering new exercises is more than just a physical achievement; it's a profound route to boosting your self-esteem and fostering a sense of personal accomplishment. Each time you learn a new movement or reach a new milestone in your chair exercise routine, you're not just improving your physical capabilities but also reinforcing your belief in your abilities. This empowerment is especially significant as we age. The aging process can often bring a sense of diminished capacity, but engaging in and mastering new physical activities can counteract this perception. Regardless of age, it reminds you of your growth potential and bolsters your self-confidence. When you gain confidence in one aspect of your life, it can also positively impact other areas. Feeling confident can motivate you to confront difficulties with a positive attitude.

Moreover, the physical improvements you experience—increased strength, better balance, and greater flexibility—are crucial in enhancing your functional independence. Imagine the activities that comprise your daily routine, such as walking up a flight of stairs, carrying groceries, or even bending down to tie your shoes. These tasks, which can become more challenging with age, can be performed more efficiently and safely as you build physical strength and agility through your exercise regimen. This functional independence is critical to maintaining an active, self-sufficient lifestyle. It allows you to continue performing everyday activities efficiently, reducing the need for assistance and fostering a sense of autonomy vital for your mental and emotional health.

Facing and overcoming the challenges presented by new and strenuous exercises can also be incredibly rewarding. When you encounter a particularly challenging routine, it might be tempting to doubt your capability. However, transforming your perspective on these challenges can make a significant difference. Instead of viewing them as obstacles, seeing them as opportunities for personal growth can change the entire experience. Overcoming challenges builds resilience, dedication, and confidence to push limits. This mindset enhances your exercise experience and prepares you to handle life's challenges with a resilient and positive outlook.

Celebrating the autonomy gained through regular exercise is equally important. Regular physical activity provides more than just health benefits; it fosters a sense of independence that can be incredibly empowering. This autonomy is especially crucial as it contradicts common stereotypes about aging, showcasing that seniors can maintain vigorous and autonomous lives. Emphasizing the significance of this independence serves as a personal triumph and an inspiration to others in your community. It demonstrates that staying active is possible and beneficial at any age, encouraging a broader cultural appreciation for health and independence among seniors.

The journey through chair exercises is much more than a path to physical health—it is a journey towards a more confident, independent, and empowered self. As you continue to engage in these exercises, remember the broader impacts of your efforts: a stronger body, a more resilient mind, and a profoundly independent spirit.

14.3 THE SOCIAL ASPECT: CONNECTING WITH OTHERS THROUGH EXERCISE

Engaging in physical activities like chair exercises benefits your physical and mental health and opens a wonderful avenue for social interaction and community building. The joy of group exercises, whether conducted in person at a local community center or online via virtual classes, extends beyond mere participation. These gatherings can transform your exercise routine into a vibrant social event, enhancing the enjoyment and benefits derived from the activity.

Group Exercise Benefits: A Gateway to Enhanced Motivation and Social Interaction

Participating in group exercises can significantly boost your motivation. There's something inherently encouraging about being part of a group that shares similar health goals. It creates an atmosphere of mutual encouragement where each member's progress and victories are celebrated, pushing everyone to persist and excel. Moreover, the structured setting of group exercises provides regularity and a sense of commitment, which can be crucial for maintaining a consistent exercise schedule. Social interactions can lead to better mental health by creating a feeling of community and belonging, which can help reduce loneliness and isolation. For seniors, who often face higher risks of social isolation, group exercises can be a vital link to the outside world and a way to maintain active social lives.

Community Engagement: Fostering Connections and Friendships Through Shared Activities

Engaging with a local or online community through exercise offers numerous opportunities to connect with like-minded individuals. You can participate in local exercise programs at community centers, which often hold classes designed specifically for seniors. These programs keep you physically active and integrate you into a community setting where friendships can flourish. For those who prefer or need to stay home, online platforms now host live exercise sessions where participants can join virtual classes and interact with instructors and fellow exercisers in real time. This can be particularly beneficial for maintaining social ties and continuing fitness routines, especially when venturing outside might not be possible.

Exercise Partners: The Benefits of Shared Motivation and Accountability

Having an exercise partner can transform your fitness routine from a solitary task into an enjoyable, shared experience. An exercise buddy provides a mutual support system where you can motivate each other to stick to your workout schedules. There's an added layer of accountability when you know someone is counting on you to show up for an exercise session. This can significantly enhance your commitment to your fitness goals. Sharing the experience can also make the time spent exercising more enjoyable, allowing for laughter and conversation, making the time pass quickly, and making the exercises feel less like a chore and more like a fun social gathering.

Inclusive Activities: Chair Exercises as a Bonding Opportunity for Friends and Family

Chair exercises can be a great way to share an activity with loved ones, regardless of age or fitness level, as they are very inclusive and accommodating. Organizing a regular exercise session with your loved ones helps you stay active and strengthens your bonds. It's a fantastic way to spend quality time together, encouraging each other and sharing the health benefits. The workout sessions can be customized to suit every individual's fitness level, ensuring that all participants feel included and none are left behind. It's about moving together, having fun, and improving everyone's health simultaneously.

In essence, the social dimensions of engaging in chair exercises enrich your exercise regimen, turning it into a more comprehensive health approach involving physical, mental, and emotional well-being, supported by a community of peers and loved ones. As this chapter closes, remember that each exercise session is more than just a moment for physical health; it's a chance to connect, share, and grow with others, enhancing the joy and benefits of your fitness journey. In the upcoming chapter, we will discuss effective methods for sustaining your enriched exercise routine, ensuring that it continues to be a lively and essential aspect of your daily life.

CHAPTER FIFTEEN

CREATING A ROUTINE THAT LASTS

I magine your daily routine as a garden. Consistent physical activity is essential for the well-being of your body and mind, just like a garden needs regular tending to thrive. Establishing a routine of chair exercises isn't just about enhancing physical fitness; it's about cultivating a lifestyle that nourishes your well-being each day. This chapter is dedicated to transforming your chair exercises from occasional activities into integral parts of your daily life, ensuring that the seeds you plant today yield health and vitality well into the future.

15.1 DAILY HABITS FOR LONG-TERM SUCCESS

Consistency is Key

The cornerstone of any successful fitness regimen is consistency. Just as a plant needs water regularly to thrive, your body needs regular movement to maintain and improve its function. Integrating chair exercises into your daily routine is critical to achieving sustained health benefits such as improved strength, balance, and flexibility. Daily physical activity has been proven to be beneficial for mental health as it helps promote clear thinking and reduce stress. This is particularly important as we age and face increasingly complex challenges.

To build this consistency, start by setting a specific time each day for your exercise. Whether it's first thing in the morning, a break during your afternoon, or a wind-down sequence before bedtime, having a set time slots for your fitness routine in your daily schedule makes it as routine as having your morning cup of coffee. This regularity helps form a habit that, once established, becomes second nature. The key is persistence. Initially, it might require a conscious effort to stick to your scheduled exercise times. Still, over time, just like any daily habit, it becomes integrated into the rhythm of your life.

Routine Integration

Integrating exercise into your daily routine can also mean associating it with other regular activities to create a seamless flow in your day. For instance, consider coupling your exercise routine with another daily habit, like watching your favorite morning show or listening to a daily podcast. This pairing can make the exercise feel like a natural part of your routine rather than a separate task to check off your list.

Additionally, consider the layout of your living space. To help you stay motivated to exercise, keep your workout chair in a visible and easily accessible spot. This way, you'll be reminded of your exercise routine and more likely to stick to it. Visual cues play a decisive role in habit formation; just seeing your exercise area can prompt you to engage in your daily workout.

Small Changes, Big Impact

Small, incremental changes are often more sustainable than ambitious overhauls, which can be daunting and challenging to maintain when establishing a lasting exercise routine. Start with short, manageable sessions, even if it's just five to ten minutes a day. As these become a habitual part of your day, gradually increase the duration or intensity of your workouts. This approach helps build endurance gently and adapts your body to new levels of activity without overwhelming it. Small daily increments lead to significant long-term health improvements, reinforcing the physical and mental benefits of your exercise routine.

Accountability Partners

Starting a fitness journey can often feel like a solitary experience. However, having a companion to share the journey with can significantly improve your dedication and enjoyment. An accountability partner—be it a friend, family member, or a member of an online community—can provide motivational support and encouragement. Sharing your goals with someone can boost your chances of achieving them since you feel accountable to someone who supports and encourages you and who may also be motivated by your progress.

Regular check-ins with your accountability partner can be a great way to stay on track. These can be quick daily texts or calls, weekly emails, or monthly meetings to share progress and setbacks. Knowing that you'll report your progress can push you to stick to your routine, and supporting someone else in their journey can boost your motivation and provide a sense of purpose and connection.

Visual Element: Routine Tracker

To aid in building your daily exercise habit, consider using a routine tracker. This simple chart or calendar can help you plan and record your exercise sessions, visually representing your consistency and progress. Mark each day you complete your exercise and watch as your activity streak grows. This tool not only serves as a record of your dedication but also as a motivational booster. Seeing a visual reminder of all the work you've put in can be incredibly satisfying and spur you to keep going, even when motivation is low.

15.2 MIXING IT UP: HOW TO KEEP CHAIR EXERCISES FRESH AND ENGAGING

It's crucial to stick to a consistent workout routine. Still, it's also essential to switch things up and make it enjoyable to avoid losing motivation and enthusiasm. Adding diversity to your workout routine goes beyond just increasing the fun factor; it also helps activate distinct muscle groups and body systems, enhancing your overall physical fitness and preventing stagnation in your workouts. Imagine your exercise routine as a colorful tapestry. Each thread represents a different form of movement, and the more varied the threads, the more vibrant and robust the tapestry becomes.

One effective way to weave this variety into your routine is by designating weekly theme days. For instance, consider Monday as 'Muscle Monday,' dedicated to strength training exercises focusing on different muscle groups using resistance bands or light weights. Transition to 'Tai Chi Tuesday,' where you focus on gentle, flowing movements emphasizing balance and flexibility. Midweek brings 'Wellness Wednesday,' concentrating on exercises that enhance cardiovascular health, like seated marching or arm cycling. As the week winds down, 'Flexibility Friday' can be your day to engage in stretches and flexibility exercises that help keep your joints and muscles supple. This themed approach not only categorizes your workouts in a fun, memorable way but also ensures a holistic approach to fitness that touches on all aspects of physical health.

Challenging yourself is also crucial in maintaining an engaging exercise routine. Setting up monthly challenges can be a great way to push your limits within safe boundaries. For example, aim to increase the duration of your 'Seated March' from five to ten minutes by the end of the month or aim to complete a set number of arm raises each week. These challenges should be tailored to your current fitness level and designed to encourage slight pushes in endurance and strength, fostering a sense of achievement and progression in your fitness journey.

Keeping an exercise diary is another invaluable tool in this process. This diary goes beyond simply tracking your exercises; it's about noting how you feel during and after each session, what works best for you, and what doesn't. Did a particular session leave you feeling rejuvenated? Or a specific movement was less comfortable than you'd hoped. Recording these observations can provide insights into how your body responds to different activities, allowing you to fine-tune your routine for maximum benefit and enjoyment. Over time, this diary will become a personalized feedback loop, offering a detailed understanding of your fitness journey and helping you make informed decisions about future exercise choices.

Incorporating these strategies into your chair exercise routine transforms your daily fitness activities into a dynamic, enjoyable, and richly rewarding part of your life. Each day brings a new focus, each week a new challenge, and your ongoing observations and adjustments ensure that your exercise routine remains tailored to your evolving needs and preferences. This approach keeps your body guessing and growing and keeps your mind engaged and enthusiastic about your path to wellness.

15.3 SETTING AND ADJUSTING GOALS OVER TIME

Creating goals is akin to plotting a course on a map during a voyage. You might know your destination, but the path you chart needs to be straightforward and adaptable, responding to the winds and the waves that might steer you slightly off course. In the realm of chair exercises, setting goals using the SMART framework— Specific, Measurable, Achievable, Relevant, and Time-bound— provides a structured way to ensure your fitness objectives are clear and within reach. For instance, rather than a vague goal like "get stronger," a SMART goal would be "to increase the duration of my seated leg lifts from one minute to three minutes over the next month." This goal is specific (increasing leg lift duration), measurable (from one to three minutes), achievable (a realistic increment), relevant (strengthening key leg muscles), and time-bound (one month).

Maintaining the vitality of your goals requires regular review and adjustment—a process not unlike pruning a plant to encourage growth. Every month, take time to reflect on your goals. Assess your progress and consider any new variables in your life, such as changes in health, motivation, or even seasonal changes that might affect your activity levels. Conducting periodic appraisals helps you adjust and fine-tune your goals to ensure they align with your current skills and ambitions. For example, suppose you've achieved a particular goal earlier than expected. In that case, you might decide to extend that goal or add a new challenge. Conversely, scaling back temporarily might be necessary to avoid discouragement if a goal becomes unattainable due to health issues.

Celebration plays a crucial role in sustaining motivation. Each time you reach a milestone, big or small, take a moment to celebrate. This could be anything from achieving a week-long streak of daily exercises to mastering a new routine that you found challenging initially. Celebrating these victories does more than feel good; it reinforces your commitment to your fitness journey and can significantly boost your morale. Consider rewarding yourself with non-material rewards, such as an extra half-hour of your favorite TV show or a relaxing bath. These celebrations highlight your progress and remind you that every effort contributes to a larger picture of improved health and enhanced quality of life.

Adapting to change is an inevitable part of life, particularly as we age. Your exercise routine and goals must be flexed as your life is. If you encounter a new health challenge, consult your healthcare provider to understand how to adjust your exercise regimen. Similarly, changes in living situations or even seasonal changes might necessitate a shift in how and when you exercise. Remain open to these changes and view them as opportunities to tailor your fitness routine more closely to your current lifestyle. This adaptability ensures that your exercise routine remains practical and enjoyable and continues to meet your evolving health needs effectively.

In wrapping up this chapter on setting and adjusting goals over time, we've navigated through the essential practices of creating clear, achievable targets, regularly assessing and recalibrating these targets, celebrating achievements to boost motivation, and staying adaptable to life's inevitable changes. These practices are pivotal in maintaining a routine and a thriving lifestyle that adapts to your needs and goals over time. As we move forward, we'll explore how leveraging technology can further support and enhance your fitness journey, integrating modern tools to keep you engaged and on track with your health objectives.

CHAPTER SIXTEEN

LEVERAGING TECHNOLOGY FOR SUPPORT

Technology's integration into our routines has impacted various areas of our lives. It can enhance our health and fitness exercise routines. Imagine technology as a complex web of gadgets and applications and as a personal assistant that helps keep your exercise routine on track. For seniors, embracing technology can often seem daunting. Yet, it offers many tools designed to make life easier, more connected, and healthier. This chapter explores easy ways to seamlessly incorporate digital tools into your daily routine, helping you achieve your fitness goals, track your progress, and enjoy the journey.

16.1 FITNESS APPS AND TRACKERS: YOUR DIGITAL COMPANIONS

App Selection: Choosing Senior-Friendly Fitness Apps

Navigating the vast landscape of fitness apps can be overwhelming, so selecting those tailored to meet your needs and preferences is essential. When searching for applications, prioritize those with an intuitive interface, legible text, and simple navigation. The ideal fitness app for seniors should provide exercise tutorials you can follow at your own pace, reminders to keep you on schedule, and tracking features that monitor your progress over time. Some apps are even designed with voice commands and audio descriptions, which can be particularly helpful if you struggle with small screens or touch interfaces.

When selecting an app, consider what you want to achieve with your chair exercises. Are you focusing on increasing flexibility, building strength, or improving cardiovascular health? There are apps specific to each of these goals. For instance, apps like 'Silver-Sneakers GO' are designed with seniors in mind and provide guided workouts, progress tracking, and customizable exercise plans. Reading reviews and possibly trying out a few free apps can help you find the best match for your fitness journey.

Wearable Trackers: Monitoring Your Health on the Go

Wearable fitness trackers are another fantastic tool for providing insights into your physical activities and health. Gadgets such as Fitbit, Garmin, or Apple Watch can monitor your heart rate, step count, sleep cycle, and even blood oxygen levels. As we age, it becomes increasingly beneficial to have access to up-to-date information about our physical condition, as it empowers us to gain a better understanding of our health and make informed decisions to enhance our overall wellness.

For example, if you're focusing on cardiovascular health, a tracker that monitors heart rate and suggests optimal heart rate zones for fitness activities can be incredibly helpful. This information allows you to adjust the intensity of your workouts to stay within a safe range, maximizing benefits while minimizing risks. Additionally, many of these devices come with fall detection and emergency SOS features, offering an added layer of security that can be comforting if you live alone.

Privacy Considerations: Safeguarding Your Information

While the benefits of fitness apps and trackers are clear, it's crucial to consider privacy and the security of your personal information. It's always a good idea to review the privacy policies of any application or device you plan to use to understand how your data will be collected, utilized, and safeguarded. Opt for apps and devices with robust security features and transparent privacy policies.

If you need clarification on any terms or settings, feel free to ask a family member or a tech-savvy friend for help. To ensure the safety of your data, it is advisable to create strong and distinct passwords for your accounts. You can also secure your data by enabling two-factor authentication wherever it is available.

Tech Savvy: Becoming Comfortable with Technology

Becoming tech-savvy might seem daunting, but it's more about taking small steps than mastering complex skills overnight. Start with the basics: learning how to set up and use your fitness tracker or navigating the features of your chosen app. Suppose you're a senior who wants to become more tech-savvy. In that case, you may find the free or low-cost courses available at local community centers and libraries helpful. These courses provide personalized support and hands-on experience, which can make the learning process less daunting.

Many apps and devices also offer tutorials, FAQs, and customer support hotlines. Utilize these resources whenever you're in doubt. Remember, every tech expert started as a beginner, and the more you use these tools, the more intuitive they will become. Embracing technology enhances your ability to maintain an active lifestyle. It connects you with new ways of managing your health and well-being in the digital age.

16.2 FINDING ONLINE SUPPORT GROUPS AND VIRTUAL CLASSES

The digital age has transformed how we connect and interact, bringing a world of opportunities to our fingertips. Online fitness communities and virtual classes provide a wealth of resources for seniors who wish to stay active and continue leading a healthy lifestyle. Some online platforms offer home-based workout routines and the chance to interact with others who share the same health and wellness objectives.

Joining an online fitness community can significantly enhance your motivation. Performing a routine on your own is one thing, but being aware that you are part of a more extensive community striving towards common objectives is another. These communities often offer a mix of encouragement, competition, and accountability that can be highly motivating. You can participate in challenges, celebrate each other's successes, and even share tips and advice. This sense of camaraderie and support is crucial, especially on days when your motivation might be waning. Furthermore, many seniors find that being part of such groups helps them stay committed to their fitness goals, as they look forward to interacting with their peers and trainers online.

Virtual chair exercise classes are another fantastic resource that has gained popularity, especially given the recent shifts towards more home-based activities. Qualified instructors usually lead these classes, and they help you perform each exercise correctly and safely. They guide you through the movements to ensure you get the most out of each workout. To find these classes, you can start by checking with local fitness centers or community groups; many have adapted to offer online sessions. Additionally, websites like YouTube have many video tutorials you can follow. Look for classes that match your fitness level and goals, and make sure that the instructor explains each movement clearly, ideally with modifications for different levels of mobility.

Sharing your milestones and success stories within these online platforms can be incredibly rewarding. Not only does this act of sharing keep you motivated, but it also inspires others. It could be something as simple as achieving a new fitness goal, mastering a challenging exercise, or noticing improvements in flexibility and balance. Sharing these achievements can inspire others in the community to strive for their goals. It also fosters a deeper connection with your peers as you support and celebrate each other's progress.

However, it's essential to navigate these online spaces safely. Keeping your personal information safe while participating in online forums or classes is necessary. When using online platforms, it's essential to stick to secure and trustworthy ones. Additionally, it's best to avoid sharing personal information like your financial details or home address. Be aware of misinformation; always verify the credentials of the people you interact with and the advice you choose to follow. If something doesn't feel right, it's essential to trust your instincts and seek advice from trusted sources or professionals.

When you make use of digital resources to aid your fitness journey, not only do you enhance your own experience, but you also become a valuable contributor to a community that values mutual support and collective knowledge. This connectivity enhances your physical health and social interactions, making the pursuit of health a more joyful and communal experience.

As this chapter concludes, remember the vast resources available through technology. From the support and camaraderie of online communities to the convenience and guidance of virtual classes, these tools offer powerful ways to enhance your fitness journey. The connections you make and the knowledge you gain can significantly enrich your path towards a healthier, more active lifestyle. As we progress, we'll explore additional strategies to keep you motivated and engaged in your fitness goals, ensuring that each step is supported and meaningful.

CHAPTER SEVENTEEN
CONTINUING YOUR JOURNEY BEYOND THE CHAIR

I magine the newfound freedom that comes with increased mobility and strength. It's like opening a door to a world brimming with possibilities that seemed slightly out of reach before. This chapter is about crossing that threshold, translating the gains from your dedicated chair exercise routine into vibrant, life-enhancing activities. It's about taking those movements from the safety and comfort of your chair and integrating them into the vast array of daily activities and new adventures life offers.

17.1 FROM CHAIR TO LIFE: TRANSLATING EXERCISE INTO EVERYDAY ACTIVITIES

Functional Fitness: Enhancing Daily Performance

Functional fitness is based on the concept that the physical exercises one engages in should improve the ease and safety with which they perform their daily activities. The strength, flexibility, and balance you cultivate through your chair exercises are not just fitness metrics; they enhance your ability to perform daily tasks. For instance, the core strength you build helps stabilize your movements when you bend to pick something off the floor, reducing the risk of falls. Similarly, the enhanced arm and shoulder strength from resistance band exercises can make lifting groceries or carrying a grandchild effortless.

Consider how the leg lifts and seated marches have toned your muscles and improved your endurance. These improvements make extended periods of walking or standing more manageable and less tiring. Even activities like climbing stairs have become safer and quicker. This direct translation of exercise into improved daily function is a testament to the value of your ongoing commitment to chair exercises.

New Opportunities: Exploring Beyond Previous Limits

As your physical capabilities expand, so does the horizon of activities available to you. Many seniors find that enhanced fitness levels open up opportunities to engage in hobbies and activities that were previously not feasible. Whether gardening now seems less daunting because you can squat and bend more efficiently or playing with your grandchildren at the park, the energy and mobility you gain turn these activities from challenges into joys.

This newfound vigor can also inspire you to travel more—perhaps walking tours that once seemed too exhausting are now inviting. Being able to walk, stand, and carry items with ease can instill a sense of confidence in one's ability to explore new places, which in turn can add a great deal of richness and adventure to one's life.

Lifestyle Integration: Making Physical Activity a Natural Part of Your Day

Incorporating regular physical activity into your daily routine involves developing a habit of moving naturally throughout the day.

This could be as simple as walking to the nearby store instead of driving or taking the stairs instead of the elevator. Each decision to move adds up, contributing to your overall health and fitness.

Another effective way to integrate more activity into your day is through incidental exercise. This involves turning routine activities into opportunities for movement. For example, while waiting for the kettle to boil, you might perform a series of calf raises or balance on one foot to practice stability. These moments can quickly become a routine part of your day, significantly boosting your activity level without requiring dedicated exercise time.

Adaptive Adventures: Inspirational Stories of Active Seniors

Many seniors have transformed their lives through fitness, engaging in adventures that reflect their passions and dreams. Take, for instance, Clara, a 78-year-old who, after strengthening her legs and improving her balance through chair yoga, decided to fulfill her lifelong dream of hiking through the national parks. Or consider James, whose improved upper body strength allowed him to return to his love for swimming, now competing in senior swim meets.

These stories are not just tales of physical accomplishment; they are powerful reminders of improved fitness's profound impact on one's quality of life. They inspire, showing that age and past limitations need not define the scope of your ambitions. Whether returning to a cherished pastime or discovering a new passion, the fitness you build in your chair can be the key to a more active and fulfilling life.

Visual Element: Adaptive Adventure Map

Consider creating an 'Adaptive Adventure Map to inspire your own adventures.' This can be a simple visual representation, like a bulletin board or digital collage, where you pin activities and destinations you wish to explore. Each pin can represent a goal; as you achieve each one, you can mark it as complete. This map is both a planning tool and a motivational visual, helping you visualize and achieve your post-exercise goals.

17.2 EXPLORING NEW HOBBIES WITH RENEWED ENERGY

As you cultivate your physical health through chair exercises, a delightful opportunity arises to channel your renewed energy into exploring new hobbies. Participating in hobbies and pastimes that align with your passions can tremendously improve your well-being by giving you a mental boost and chances for social engagement. Think of hobbies as the seasoning in the recipe of life; they add flavor, color, and zest, transforming everyday routines into rich, fulfilling experiences.

Hobby Ideas: Diverse Options for Enriched Living

One of the joys of improved physical fitness is the ability to partake in a broader range of activities. Dance classes, for instance, are excellent for those who enjoy moving to music and can be a terrific way to maintain flexibility, balance, and endurance; for those intrigued by the arts, painting or pottery classes offer a creative outlet that also fine-tunes motor skills and cognitive function. Photography, particularly nature photography, not only fosters artistic expression but encourages outdoor activity, which is beneficial for mental and physical health. Birdwatching combines gentle walks in nature with the mentally stimulating activity of identifying different species, perfect for those who appreciate wildlife and tranquil settings.

Another engaging option is cooking classes that focus on nutritious recipes. These can be especially rewarding, combining learning new culinary skills with the practical benefits of enhancing your diet.

For those with a knack for technology, computer classes can open up the digital world, offering skills that range from essential computer use to more advanced lessons in social media or digital photography, keeping you connected and engaged with modern communication tools.

Learning and Growth: Cognitive and Emotional Enhancements

Learning new skills has profound benefits on cognitive health, particularly for seniors. Engaging in new activities stimulates the brain, enhancing memory, problem-solving, and critical thinking. This mental engagement is crucial for maintaining cognitive vitality and can even slow the progression of age-related cognitive decline. Furthermore, the satisfaction that comes from mastering a new skill can boost self-esteem and overall well-being.

Emotionally, hobbies provide a sense of accomplishment and pleasure. They break the monotony of daily routines, infuse life with excitement, and offer something to look forward to each day. Whether it's the pride of crafting something with your hands or the thrill of capturing a perfect photograph, hobbies enrich your emotional world, bringing joy and a sense of achievement.

Community Classes: Social Connections and Skill Building

Community classes are a fantastic resource for exploring new interests while meeting like-minded individuals. Many community centers, libraries, and colleges offer various courses that are often senior-friendly and sometimes even specifically designed for older adults. The classes facilitate connections and cultivate community among individuals with shared interests.

Participating in these classes can significantly enhance your social life, which is vital for emotional health. Attending community classes can be a great way to combat loneliness and isolation, as it offers opportunities for social interaction, emotional support, and a greater sense of belonging. You can feel secure in these settings while learning and developing your skills. The instructors are experienced in working with people of different skill levels, so you can advance at your own pace without feeling rushed or overwhelmed.

Barriers to Entry: Overcoming Hurdles to Engagement

Despite the many benefits, taking up new hobbies can sometimes seem daunting. Many people face obstacles such as the fear of failing, a sense of not belonging, or feeling lost when trying to achieve their goals. Nevertheless, with appropriate tactics, it is possible to overcome these challenges.

Start by choosing low-risk activities that require minimal investment. This will reduce the pressure to excel and allow you to explore interests without significant commitment. Many community centers offer free trial classes, a great way to test a hobby before committing. If fear of the unknown is holding you back, consider inviting a friend to join you. Tackling a new activity with a companion can alleviate anxiety and enhance the enjoyment of the experience.

Finally, remember that everyone was a beginner at some point. Be patient with yourself and allow time to learn and grow. Instructors and fellow hobbyists are generally supportive and understanding, and many are likely to have been in your shoes at one time. Embracing this supportive environment can help you overcome initial fears and fully enjoy learning something new.

By exploring new hobbies, you enrich your life with enjoyable activities and contribute to your physical, cognitive, and emotional health. Each new skill learned and each connection made adds another layer of depth to your life, proving that growth and discovery are always within reach, no matter your age.

17.3 VOLUNTEERING: GIVING BACK WITH YOUR GAINED STRENGTH AND MOBILITY

Volunteering is a beautiful bridge that connects experience with action, knowledge with sharing, and fitness with community service. As you grow stronger and more mobile, you might find yourself looking for meaningful ways to utilize these gains. Volunteering allows you to give back to your community in impactful ways and enriches your life with purpose and connection. It's a reciprocal relationship where your contributions help build a stronger community. In return, you experience the profound joy and satisfaction of service.

A vast array of volunteering opportunities are particularly well-suited to seniors. These roles can range from active tasks like helping in community gardens, which can be excellent for those who have regained or maintained their physical mobility through chair exercises, to more passive roles such as knitting blankets for newborns in hospitals or making calls for a telecare service that supports isolated individuals. For those who enjoy social interaction, volunteering at local museums or as tour guides at community parks offers a great way to stay active and engage with people regularly. These activities keep you moving and provide the social perks of interacting with a diverse group of people, from fellow volunteers to community members of all ages.

Volunteering can also profoundly impact your sense of purpose and overall well-being. Engaging in volunteer work can instill a strong sense of purpose by contributing to the community and knowing that your efforts are helping to make a difference. This can be especially meaningful during retirement, as it helps fill the space once occupied by a career or daily job, giving structure to your days and a reason to stay active and involved. It's not uncommon for volunteers to express feelings of renewed purpose and a greater sense of belonging to a community, as regular interactions and shared goals foster a deep connection with others.

Furthermore, the impact of your volunteer work can be significant, regardless of the scale. Organizations can significantly benefit from seniors' vast experience and distinct skills. For example, those who have cultivated a garden for years could provide invaluable advice and hands-on help in community or school gardens, teaching younger generations the importance of sustainable practices and healthy eating. Similarly, those who have honed communication skills over a lifetime could offer mentoring to young people or lead workshops. Each act of volunteering, no matter how small it might seem, contributes to a larger tapestry of community support and development, making a tangible difference in the lives of others.

Finding the right volunteering opportunity involves carefully considering your interests, physical capabilities, and what you hope to get from the experience. Start by identifying your passion—is it education, health, the environment, or perhaps the arts? Volunteering can be a great way to give back to your community. You may consider contacting local community centers, non-profit organizations, or religious groups to find opportunities that match your interests and skills. They can assist you in finding a volunteer role that is both fulfilling and rewarding. It's also worth considering how much time you can commit to volunteering. Some roles may require a regular weekly commitment. In contrast, others might be more flexible, involving one-off events or seasonal activities.

Additionally, check for any physical requirements that may be involved, especially for more active roles. Choosing an opportunity that matches your mobility level is important to ensure you can perform tasks safely and comfortably. Many organizations are accommodating and can tailor roles to fit individual abilities and strengths. Don't hesitate to discuss your needs and expectations with the volunteer coordinator—open communication will help ensure that the role is a good fit, allowing you to contribute effectively without compromising your health or well-being.

Engaging in volunteer work as you grow older is not just about giving back to the community but also about continuing to enrich your life through active participation and social engagement. By choosing roles that align with your interests and abilities, you ensure that your volunteer experiences are fulfilling and enjoyable, enhancing your life and the lives of those around you.

17.4 SETTING NEW HORIZONS: GOALS BEYOND CHAIR EXERCISES

In the golden years of life, it's crucial not just to think about maintaining health and mobility but to envision a future that expands in richness and depth. The encouragement to set long-term health and wellness goals is more than a suggestion—it's an invitation to dream bigger and live fully, well beyond the confines of chair exercises. These aspirations should focus on maintaining physical capabilities and embracing a lifestyle that celebrates active aging. This lifelong wellness journey is about adding years to life and, most importantly, adding life to those years.

Long-term goals might include:

- Hiking a new trail each year.
- Dancing at a grandchild's wedding.
- Even starting a small garden that you tend to daily.

These goals anchor you in a mindset that views aging as an adventure to be welcomed with enthusiasm rather than a time of inevitable decline. The objective is to cultivate a lifestyle where activity is intertwined with daily living. This ensures that each day is lived with vigor and purpose.

Continuous learning and embracing new fitness challenges are pivotal to staying on this path. The world of health and fitness is ever-evolving, with new research and strategies emerging that can enhance your quality of life. Staying informed about these developments keeps your routine fresh. It empowers you with the knowledge to make the best decisions for your health. Engaging with new information could mean subscribing to a health newsletter, joining a wellness workshop, or simply swapping tips with friends who prioritize their health. This ongoing educational journey ensures that your approach to health and fitness remains dynamic and tailored to your evolving needs.

Moreover, your goals should be living entities, expected to grow and change as you do. Periodically reviewing and adapting these goals ensures they remain aligned with your current health status, interests, and realistic opportunities. You may have started with goals focused on physical health, but now you want to include more social activities. Adjusting your goals to join a walking group or a dance class reflects this growth. It's about recalibrating your ambitions to match your current reality, ensuring that your goals continue to challenge yet inspire you.

Finally, consider the legacy you wish to leave. This isn't just about the memories or possessions you pass on but about fostering a culture of health and activity within your family and community. Embodying a lifestyle that values health and active living inspires others to follow in your footsteps. Whether it's your children, grandchildren, or neighbors, showing that age is not a barrier to living actively encourages others to adopt the same mindset. This legacy of health is the most profound gift you can offer, as it promises to improve the lives of others well beyond your own.

Through setting expansive long-term goals, embracing continuous learning, adapting your aspirations, and considering the legacy you wish to establish, you are doing more than just living; you are thriving. Each step you take in this direction enhances your life and serves as a beacon for others, proving that every day is an opportunity to grow, learn, and contribute.

Moving forward into the next chapter, we will explore additional resources that can support your journey into active aging. These tools and insights will ensure you have everything you need to implement your plans, achieve your goals, and continue setting new horizons for years.

CHAIR EXERCISES FOR SENIORS SIMPLIFIED

THE ILLUSTRATED BEGINNER'S GUIDE TO IMPROVE YOUR BALANCE AND MOBILITY WITH EASY YOGA AND STRENGTH ROUTINES

Congratulations on finishing "Chair Exercises for Seniors Simplified"!

Now that you have all the tools to live a healthier and more active life, it's time to share your newfound knowledge and help other readers find the same benefits.

By leaving your honest opinion of this book on Amazon, you'll help fellow seniors find the information they're looking for and spread the joy of chair exercise.

Thank you for your help. Chair exercising thrives when we pass on our knowledge, and you're helping us do just that.

Simply scan the QR code to leave your review:

Thank you again for being part of this journey. Keep moving and stay active!

- Your biggest fan, Insight Editions

CONCLUSION

As we draw this guide to a close, let us take a moment to reflect on the transformative journey we've embarked upon together. From those initial hesitations and physical limitations to a newfound sense of empowerment and vitality, chair exercises offer a remarkable path to enhanced well-being for seniors. These exercises are not just movements but stepping stones to a more independent and fulfilling lifestyle.

During our conversations, we have delved into the benefits of chair exercises, which are tailor-made to cater to the specific needs of seniors. These exercises provide a secure, efficient, and convenient way to enhance strength, flexibility, and balance. This is not just about fitness; it's about reclaiming the joys of an active life and the independence that comes with it.

We've shared stories and testimonials from individuals just like you, who once faced daily routines with difficulty and now celebrate life with renewed vigor. These stories are a testament to the transformative power of chair exercises, offering hope and inspiration for your own journey

RESOURCES

National Center for Biotechnology Information (NCBI). "The Effect of Chair-Based Exercise on Physical Function in Older Adults." https://www.ncbi.nlm.nih.gov/pmc/articles/PMC7920319/

Senior Helpers. "How to Create a Senior-Friendly Exercise Space at Home." https://www.seniorhelpers.com/va/stafford/resources/blogs/how-to-create-a-senior-friendly-exercise-space-at-home/

Senior Lifestyle. "Infographic: Top 10 Chair Yoga Positions for Seniors." https://www.seniorlifestyle.com/resources/blog/infographic-top-10-chair-yoga-positions-for-seniors/

American Association of Retired Persons (AARP). "5 Ways to Avoid an Exercise Injury After Age 50." https://www.aarp.org/health/healthy-living/info-2021/exercise-injury.html

Edward-Elmhurst Health. "9 Chair Exercises for Limited Mobility." https://www.eehealth.org/blog/2022/02/chair-exercises-for-limited-mobility/

WebMD. "Best Chair Exercises for Seniors." https://www.webmd.com/fitness-exercise/best-chair-exercises-for-seniors

WebMD. "Physical Fitness for People With a Visual Impairment." https://www.webmd.com/eye-health/what-to-know-about-physical-fitness-for-blind-or-low-vision-people

SilverSneakers. "Small-Space, Full-Body Workout for Seniors." https://www.silversneakers.com/blog/small-space-full-body-workout-older-adults/

Live Science."What are the Benefits of Resistance Bands?" https://www.livescience.com/benefits-of-resistance-bands

Greatist. "21 DIY Gym Equipment Projects to Make at Home." https://greatist.com/fitness/21-diy-gym-equipment-projects-make-home

National Institute on Aging (NIA). "How Older Adults Can Get Started With Exercise." https://www.nia.nih.gov/health/exercise-and-physical-activity/how-older-adults-can-get-started-exercise

SilverSneakers."8 Best Fitness Apps for Older Adults."https://www.silversneakers.com/blog/8-best-fitness-apps-for-older-adults/

American Heart Association. "Target Heart Rates Chart."https://www.heart.org/en/healthy-living/fitness/fitness-basics/target-heart-rates

National Center for Biotechnology Information (NCBI). "The Effectiveness of Dance

Interventions to Improve Older Adults' Health." https://www.ncbi.nlm.nih.gov/pmc/articles/PMC5491389/

American Council on Exercise (ACE). "Cardio Exercises for Active Agers." https://www.acefitness.org/resources/pros/expert-articles/6553/cardio-exercises-for-active-agers/

Garage Gym Reviews. "The Best Resistance Bands for Seniors (2024)." https://www.garagegymreviews.com/best-resistance-bands-for-seniors

Harvard Health Publishing, Harvard Medical School. "The Best Core Exercises for Older Adults." https://www.health.harvard.edu/staying-healthy/the-best-core-exercises-for-older-adults

Westmont Living. "Top 10 Leg Exercise for Seniors: Easy & Effective Tips." https://westmontliving.com/blog/activities/top-10-leg-exercise-for-seniors-easy-effective-tips/

VIPcare. "5 Ways to Avoid Common Exercise Injuries for Older Adults." https://getvipcare.com/blog/5-ways-to-avoid-exercise-injuries-in-older-adults/

National Center for Biotechnology Information (NCBI)."Flexibility Training and Functional Ability in Older Adults." https://www.ncbi.nlm.nih.gov/pmc/articles/PMC3503322/

American Council on Exercise (ACE)."Chair Yoga Poses | 7 Poses for Better Balance." https://www.acefitness.org/resources/everyone/blog/5478/chair-yoga-poses-7-poses-for-better-balance/

Medical News Today. "Stretching Exercises for Seniors: Back, Neck, and More." https://www.medicalnewstoday.com/articles/stretching-exercises-for-seniors

HelpGuide. "How to Exercise with Limited Mobility." https://www.helpguide.org/articles/healthy-living/chair-exercises-and-limited-mobility-fitness.htm

Medical News Today. "Chair Yoga for Seniors: Benefits and Poses for Beginners." https://www.medicalnewstoday.com/articles/chair-yoga-for-seniors

Prana Sutra. "Yoga for Seniors + 5 Breathing Exercises (Pranayama) for Older Adults." https://www.prana-sutra.com/post/yoga-pranayama-for-seniors-older-adults

Sunrise Medical. "Yoga Positions for Wheelchair Users." https://www.sunrisemedical.eu/blog/yoga-positions-wheelchair-users-1

RetireGuide. "Meditation for Seniors: Benefits & Techniques to Get Started." https://www.retireguide.com/retirement-life-leisure/healthy-aging/mental-wellness/meditation/

Arthritis Foundation. "Seated Workout Demo." https://www.arthritis.org/health-wellness/healthy-living/physical-activity/getting-started/your-exercise-solution/combined-movements/seated-workout

Sit and Be Fit. "Exercises for Osteoporosis." https://www.sitandbefit.org/exercises-for-osteoporosis/

British Heart Foundation (BHF). "5 More Easy Chair Exercises - Heart Matters." https://www.bhf.org.uk/informationsupport/heart-matters-magazine/activity/chair-based-exercises/5-more-chair-based-exercises

National Institute on Aging (NIA). "Exercising With Chronic Conditions." https://www.nia.nih.gov/health/exercise-and-physical-activity/exercising-chronic-conditions

The Note Ninjas. "7 Upper Body Exercises to Help Improve Wheelchair Mobility." https://thenoteninjas.com/blog/f/upper-body-exercises-to-help-improve-wheelchair-mobility

HUR USA. "6 Core Strength Training Exercises for Wheelchair Users." https://hurusa.com/6-core-strength-training-exercises-for-wheelchair-users/

Spinal Cord. "Fitness Equipment For Wheelchair Users - A Visual Tour." https://www.spinalcord.org/disability-products-services/fitness-equipment-for-wheelchair-users/

HelpGuide. "How to Exercise with Limited Mobility."https://www.helpguide.org/articles/healthy-living/chair-exercises-and-limited-mobility-fitness.htm

National Institute on Aging (NIA). "How Older Adults Can Get Started With Exercise." https://www.nia.nih.gov/health/exercise-and-physical-activity/how-older-adults-can-get-started-exercise

National Institute on Aging (NIA). "How Can Strength Training Build Healthier Bodies as We Age?" https://www.nia.nih.gov/news/how-can-strength-training-build-healthier-bodies-we-age

Lifeline. "14 Dumbbell & Resistance Band Exercises For Seniors." https://www.lifeline.ca/en/resources/dumbbell-and-resistance-band-exercises-for-seniors/

Cano Health. "7 Injury Prevention Exercises for Seniors." https://canohealth.com/news/blog/7-injury-prevention-exercises-for-seniors/

Better Health Channel. "Nutrition Needs When You're Over 65." https://www.betterhealth.vic.gov.au/health/healthyliving/Nutrition-needs-when-youre-over-65

National Heart, Lung, and Blood Institute (NHLBI), NIH. "Good Hydration Linked to Healthy Aging." https://www.nhlbi.nih.gov/news/2023/good-hydration-linked-healthy-aging

A Place for Mom. "20 Nutritious and Easy Recipes for Senior Nutrition." https://www.aplaceformom.com/caregiver-resources/articles/easy-recipes-for-senior-nutrition

Healthline. "A Definitive Guide to Supplements for Healthy Aging." https://www.healthline.com/nutrition/a-definitive-guide-to-supplements-for-healthy-aging

National Institute on Aging (NIA). "A Good Night's Sleep."https://www.nia.nih.gov/health/sleep/good-nights-sleep

National Center for Biotechnology Information (NCBI). "Effects of Chair-Based

Resistance Band Exercise on Physical Function in Older Adults." https://www. ncbi.nlm.nih.gov/pmc/articles/PMC9969069/

HelpGuide. "Sleep and Aging: Sleep Tips for Older Adults." https://www.helpguide. org/articles/sleep/how-to-sleep-well-as-you-age.htm

Sleep Foundation. "How Can Exercise Affect Sleep?" https://www.sleepfoundation. org/physical-activity/exercise-and-sleep

National Institute on Aging (NIA). "How Older Adults Can Get Started With Exercise." https://www.nia.nih.gov/health/exercise-and-physical-activity/how-older-adults-can-get-started-exercise

National Center for Biotechnology Information (NCBI). "The Effectiveness, Suitability, and Sustainability of Non-Pharmacological Methods for Seniors." https:// www.ncbi.nlm.nih.gov/pmc/articles/PMC6842175/

SilverSneakers. "5 Warm-Up Exercises for Seniors: Tips from the Experts." https:// www.silversneakers.com/blog/warm-up-exercise/

PT Health. "How to Tell the Difference Between Good and Bad Pain." https://www. pthealth.ca/blog/how-to-tell-the-difference-between-good-and-bad-pain/

National Center for Biotechnology Information (NCBI). "The Importance of Physical Activity Exercise among Older Adults." https://www.ncbi.nlm.nih.gov/pmc/arti cles/PMC6304477/

Better Health Channel. "Physical Activity - How to Get Active When You Are Busy." https://www.betterhealth.vic.gov.au/health/healthyliving/Physical-activity-how-to-get-active-when-you-are-busy

Cleveland Clinic. "How SMART Fitness Goals Can Help You Get Healthier." https:// health.clevelandclinic.org/smart-fitness-goals

Independence Now (INNOW). "Adaptive Fitness: Wellness for People with Disabilities through Exercise." https://www.innow.org/2023/09/07/adaptive-fitness-well ness-for-people-with-disabilities-through-exercise/

SilverSneakers. "8 Best Fitness Apps for Older Adults." https://www.silversneakers. com/blog/8-best-fitness-apps-for-older-adults/

AgeWell Senior Fitness. "Best Wearable Fitness Trackers for Seniors - Essential Guide for Older Adults." [https://agewellseniorfitness.com/best-wearable-fitness-trackers-for-seniors-essential-guide-for-older-adults/

CyberGuy. "How to Stop Health and Fitness Apps from Using Your Private Data." https://cyberguy.com/security/how-to-stop-health-and-fitness-apps-from-using-your-private-data/

Arizona Non-Medical Home Care Association (AZNHA). "Why Are Virtual Exercise Classes a Good Option for Seniors?" https://aznha.org/why-are-virtual-exercise-classes-a-good-option-for-seniors/

National Center for Biotechnology Information (NCBI). "The Relationship Between

Physical Activity, Physical Fitness, and Health in Older Adults." https://www.ncbi.nlm.nih.gov/pmc/articles/PMC9853435/

The New York Times. "Be Here Now: How to Exercise Mindfully." https://www.nytimes.com/2022/01/28/well/move/exercise-mindfulness.html

Mayo Clinic. "Depression and Anxiety: Exercise Eases Symptoms." https://www.mayoclinic.org/diseases-conditions/depression/in-depth/depression-and-exercise/art-20046495

University of Missouri News. "Group Exercise Boosts Physical, Mental Health for Older Adults, MU Study Finds." https://showme.missouri.edu/2022/group-exercise-boosts-physical-mental-health-for-older-adults-mu-study-finds/

SilverSneakers. "Functional Exercises for Seniors: Improve Balance and More." https://www.silversneakers.com/blog/functional-fitness-the-silversneakers-guide/

Health.com. "Hobbies Like Gardening, Fishing Can Boost Your Brain Health." https://www.health.com/hobbies-for-cognitive-health-7970193

SilverSneakers. "Volunteering for Seniors: 10 Great Opportunities." https://www.silversneakers.com/blog/volunteer-opportunities/

National Institute on Aging (NIA). "How Older Adults Can Get Started With Exercise." https://www.nia.nih.gov/health/exercise-and-physical-activity/how-older-adults-can-get-started-exercise

www.ingramcontent.com/pod-product-compliance
Lightning Source LLC
Chambersburg PA
CBHW050221270326
41914CB00003BA/517

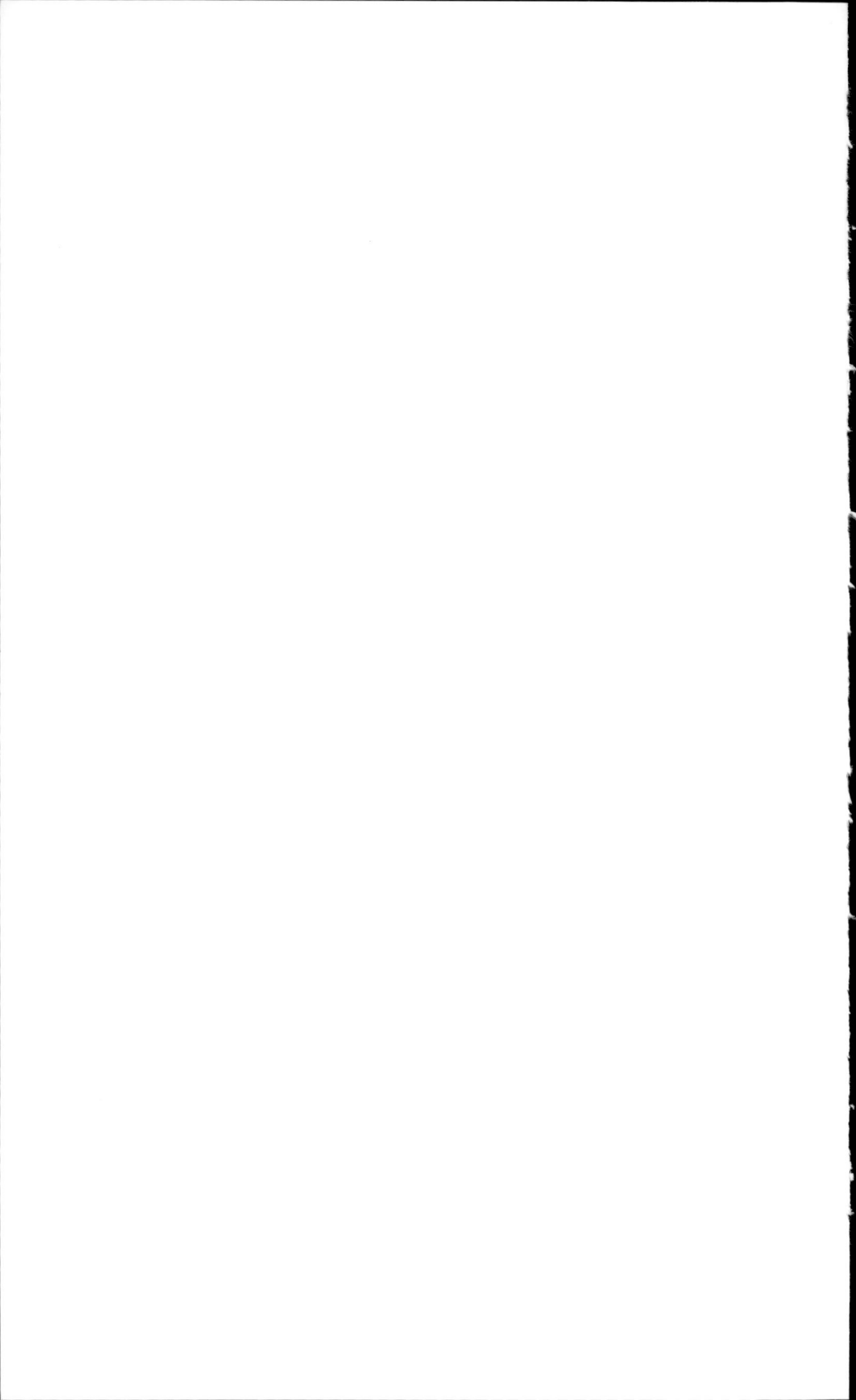